The Anti-Inflammatory Restoration Diet

By

Anthony

Nourishing Foods to Calm Inflammation and Renew Vitality

Copyright © 2024 by Anthony Richard

All rights reserved. No part of this publication may be reproduced, distributed, or transmitted in any form or by any means, including photocopying, recording, or other electronic or mechanical methods, without the prior written permission of the publisher, except in the case of brief quotations embodied in critical reviews and certain other noncommercial uses permitted by copyright law.

Table of Contents

INTRODUCTION: INFLAMMATION AND ITS IMPACT ON HEALTH
- Types of Inflammation
- The Role of Diet and Lifestyle
- The Gut Connection, Inflammatory Responses and Diseases
- The Basics of Anti-Inflammatory Eating
- Foods and Oils to Avoid
- Benefits of Adopting an Anti-Inflammatory Diet
- Kitchen Tools and Gadgets for Easy Meal Preparation
- Tips for Organizing Your Kitchen Space
- Meal Planning and Preparation

Easy Recipes for Busy Mornings
- Scrambled Eggs or Tofu with Spinach
- Quinoa Breakfast Bowl
- Breakfast Tacos
- Green Smoothie with Kale
- Buckwheat Pancakes
- Veggie & Hummus Wrap
- Quinoa Bowl with Dried Apricots
- Cottage Cheese or Dairy-Free Yogurt Bowl
- Breakfast Burrito
- Oatmeal Bowl with Poached Egg
- Whole Grain Waffles
- Veggie & Tofu Scramble

Breakfast Muffins Combo
Smoked Salmon & Cream Cheese
Tropical Smoothie Bowl
Turkey Bacon Avocado Wrap
Vegetable Frittata
Tuna Salad Wrap
Blueberry Almond Overnight Oats
Peanut Butter Banana Smoothie Bowl
Egg and Veggie Wrap
Spinach and Feta Egg Muffins
Bacon and Cheddar Egg Muffins

Breakfast Ideas for Meal Preparation

Egg Muffin Cups
Smoothie Packs
Coconut Yogurt Parfait
Breakfast Muffins
Breakfast Burrito Wraps
Steel-Cut Oats with Almond Butter
Protein-Packed Quinoa Bowl
Baked Oatmeal Squares
Avocado and Smoked Salmon Toast
Tofu Scramble Wraps
Berry and Spinach Breakfast Smoothie Packs
Bircher Muesli
Fluffy Whole Wheat Pancakes
Denver Omelet
Quinoa Breakfast Bowl
Chorizo and Egg Breakfast Burrito

Savory Cheddar Chive Waffles

Vegetarian and Vegan Options

Lentil and Walnut Meatballs
Mediterranean Quinoa Bowl
Kale and Roasted Vegetable Salad
Vegetable Soup
Chickpea Curry
Chickpea Salad
Roasted Vegetable Buddha Bowl
Lentil Soup
Tofu Stir-Fry
Eggplant and Chickpea Curry
Quinoa Stuffed Bell Peppers
Vegetable and Lentil Shepherd's Pie
Spinach and Mushroom Quesadillas
Sweet Potato and Black Bean Tacos
Zucchini Noodles with Pesto
Pudding with Berries (Vegan)
Vegan Lentil Sloppy Joes
Cauliflower and Chickpea Curry
Mushroom and Spinach Quinoa Pilaf
Vegan Chili
Stuffed Portobello Mushrooms
Tofu Scramble Breakfast Tacos
Vegan Pad Thai
Veggie and Hummus Wrap

Poultry, Meat and Potatoes

Lemon Herb Baked Chicken

Beef and Broccoli Stir-Fry
Roasted Sweet Potato Wedges
Shepherd's Pie
Turkey Meatballs with Zucchini Noodles
Herb-Roasted Turkey Breast
Honey Mustard Glazed Chicken
Mediterranean Chicken Skewers
Herb-Roasted Potatoes
Balsamic Glazed Salmon
Garlic and Herb Steak
Sweet Potato and Black Bean Hash
Mashed Cauliflower and Garlic Potatoes
Roasted Fingerling Potatoes
Greek Potato Salad
Ginger Soy Glazed Pork Chops
Turmeric Lamb Kabobs
Chili Lime Shrimp Tacos

Sauces, Condiments and Dressings

Almond Butter
Balsamic Vinaigrette
Guacamole
Taco Seasoning
Lemon Tahini Dressing
Avocado Cilantro Lime Sauce
Garlic-Herb Yogurt Sauce
Roasted Red Pepper Pesto
Lemon-Tahini Sauce
Cucumber Yogurt Sauce

- Balsamic Honey Glaze
- Green Dressing
- Spicy Mango Salsa

Fruit-Based Treats, Beverages and Herbal Teas for Hydration

- Watermelon and Mint Salad
- Green Smoothie
- Baked Apples with Cinnamon and Honey
- Lemon and Cucumber Infused Water
- Rainbow Fruit Salad
- Berry Antioxidant Smoothie
- Ginger Lemonade
- Green Tea Smoothie
- Golden Milk Latte
- Chamomile Tea
- Peppermint Tea
- Hibiscus Tea
- Ginger Turmeric Tea

28 DAYS MEAL PLAN

INDEX

INTRODUCTION: INFLAMMATION AND ITS IMPACT ON HEALTH

Inflammation is the body's natural response to injury or infection. It is a protective mechanism that helps remove harmful stimuli and initiates the healing process. However, when inflammation becomes chronic, it can lead to various health issues and exacerbate existing conditions. Chronic inflammation has been linked to diseases such as heart disease, cancer, Alzheimer's, arthritis, and autoimmune disorders.

Types of Inflammation

There are two main types of inflammation: acute and chronic. Acute inflammation is a short-term response to a specific injury or infection, characterized by redness, swelling, heat, and pain. On the other hand, chronic inflammation is a prolonged and persistent state of low-level inflammation that can last for months or even years.

The Role of Diet and Lifestyle

While inflammation is a natural bodily process, certain dietary and lifestyle factors can contribute to its development and persistence. Unhealthy eating habits, lack of physical activity, stress, and environmental toxins can all promote chronic inflammation. Conversely, a healthy diet rich in anti-inflammatory foods and an active lifestyle can help reduce inflammation and promote overall well-being.

The Gut Connection, Inflammatory Responses and Diseases

The gut plays a crucial role in regulating inflammation in the body. An imbalance in gut bacteria, also known as dysbiosis, can lead to increased inflammation and contribute to various inflammatory conditions, such as inflammatory bowel disease, rheumatoid arthritis, and even depression. Maintaining a healthy gut through a balanced diet and probiotic supplementation can help mitigate inflammatory responses and reduce the risk of related diseases.

The Basics of Anti-Inflammatory Eating

An anti-inflammatory diet emphasizes the consumption of whole, nutrient-dense foods that can help reduce inflammation in the body. This includes a variety of fruits, vegetables, whole grains, lean proteins, and healthy fats. At the same time, it limits the intake of processed foods, refined carbohydrates, and unhealthy fats, which can contribute to inflammation.

Foods and Oils to Avoid

While an anti-inflammatory diet focuses on incorporating nutrient-rich, whole foods, there are certain foods and oils that can promote inflammation and should be limited or avoided. These include:

Processed and Refined Carbohydrates Foods high in refined carbohydrates, such as white bread, pastries, crackers, and sugary snacks, can spike blood sugar levels and contribute to inflammation. These processed foods often lack fiber and nutrients and may contain unhealthy fats and additives.

Fried Foods Fried foods are typically cooked in oils heated to high temperatures, which can create trans fats and advanced glycation end products (AGEs) that drive inflammation. Examples include french fries, fried chicken, doughnuts, and other deep-fried items.

Refined Vegetable and Seed Oils Oils like corn, soybean, sunflower, and safflower oils are high in pro-inflammatory omega-6 fatty acids. These refined oils are often used in processed foods and should be replaced with healthier options like extra virgin olive oil or avocado oil.

Red and Processed Meats Red meats, especially those that are processed or cured, can promote inflammation due to their high content of saturated fats and advanced glycation end products (AGEs). Examples include bacon, sausages, hot dogs, and deli meats.

Sugary Beverages Sodas, fruit juices, and other sugary drinks are a significant source of added sugars, which can contribute to inflammation, weight gain, and other health issues. These beverages lack nutrients and can spike blood sugar levels.

Alcohol Excessive alcohol consumption can lead to inflammation and damage to various organs, including the liver, brain, and heart. Moderation is key, and it's best to avoid alcohol if you're dealing with chronic inflammatory conditions.

Artificial Sweeteners and Additives Many processed foods contain artificial sweeteners, colors, and preservatives, which can potentially contribute to inflammation and other adverse health effects.

By limiting or avoiding these inflammatory foods and oils, and focusing on a diet rich in whole, nutrient-dense foods, you can help reduce inflammation and promote overall health and well-being.

Benefits of Adopting an Anti-Inflammatory Diet

Incorporating an anti-inflammatory diet into your lifestyle can provide numerous benefits for your overall health and well-being. By reducing chronic inflammation, you can mitigate the risk of various diseases and improve your quality of life. Here are some of the key benefits of adopting an anti-inflammatory diet:

1. **Reduced Risk of Chronic Diseases**: Chronic inflammation is a significant contributing factor to the development of many diseases, including heart disease, cancer, Alzheimer's, arthritis, and autoimmune disorders. By reducing inflammation through a nutrient-

rich diet, you can lower your risk of these chronic conditions.
2. **Improved Gut Health**: An anti-inflammatory diet, rich in fiber, probiotics, and prebiotics, can support a healthy gut microbiome. This, in turn, can improve digestion, nutrient absorption, and immune function, as well as reduce the risk of inflammatory bowel diseases.
3. **Better Weight Management**: Chronic inflammation has been linked to obesity and metabolic disorders. An anti-inflammatory diet, which emphasizes nutrient-dense foods and healthy fats, can promote a balanced metabolism and support weight management efforts.
4. **Reduced Joint Pain and Arthritis Symptoms**: Inflammatory conditions like rheumatoid arthritis and osteoarthritis can cause significant joint pain and stiffness. By reducing inflammation through diet, many individuals experience relief from these symptoms and improved mobility.
5. **Improved Brain Function and Mental Health**: Inflammation has been associated with cognitive decline, depression, and other mental health issues. An anti-inflammatory diet, rich in antioxidants and omega-3 fatty acids, can support brain health and potentially reduce the risk of neurodegenerative diseases.

6. **Increased Energy Levels**: Chronic inflammation can contribute to fatigue and low energy levels. By reducing inflammation and providing your body with nutrient-dense foods, you may experience increased vitality and improved overall energy.
7. **Healthier Skin**: Inflammatory processes can contribute to skin conditions such as acne, eczema, and psoriasis. An anti-inflammatory diet may help alleviate these skin issues and promote a healthier complexion.
8. **Reduced Risk of Allergies and Asthma**: Inflammation plays a role in the development and exacerbation of allergies and asthma. Following an anti-inflammatory diet may help manage these conditions and reduce the need for medication.

Kitchen Tools and Gadgets for Easy Meal Preparation

Adopting an anti-inflammatory diet can be a lifestyle change that requires some adjustment in the kitchen. Having the right tools and gadgets can make meal preparation more efficient, enjoyable, and hassle-free. Here are some essential kitchen items that can simplify your journey to a healthier, inflammation-reducing diet:

1. **High-quality Knives**: Invest in a good set of knives, including a chef's knife, a paring knife, and a serrated knife. Sharp knives make chopping and slicing vegetables, fruits, and proteins a breeze, reducing prep time and ensuring even cutting.
2. **Vegetable Spiralizer**: This gadget transforms vegetables like zucchini, sweet potatoes, and carrots into long, noodle-like strands, providing a healthy alternative to traditional pasta.
3. **High-Speed Blender**: A powerful blender is a versatile tool for making smoothies, nut butters, dressings, and even nut milk from scratch. It helps incorporate nutrient-dense ingredients into your meals effortlessly.
4. **Mandoline Slicer**: This kitchen tool allows you to quickly and evenly slice vegetables, making it easier to prepare dishes like veggie noodles, salads, and roasted vegetable medleys.
5. **Immersion Blender**: An immersion blender is handy for blending soups, sauces, and dressings right in the pot or container, minimizing mess and simplifying cleanup.
6. **Food Processor**: A food processor can chop, slice, shred, and even knead dough for homemade breads and crusts, saving you time and effort in the kitchen.

7. **Slow Cooker or Instant Pot**: These versatile appliances allow you to prepare nutrient-dense meals with minimal effort, making it easier to incorporate more whole foods into your diet.
8. **Grill Pan or Indoor Grill**: Grilling is a healthy cooking method that can add flavor to proteins and vegetables without the need for excessive oils or fats.
9. **Spiralizer or Julienne Peeler**: These tools create long, thin strips or noodles from vegetables like zucchini, carrots, and beets, providing a fun and nutritious alternative to traditional pasta.
10. **High-Quality Pots and Pans**: Invest in a good set of pots and pans, preferably made of non-toxic materials like cast iron, stainless steel, or ceramic, to ensure even cooking and easy cleanup.

Tips for Organizing Your Kitchen Space

An organized kitchen can make meal preparation smoother, more efficient, and even encourage you to cook more often. When your space is clutter-free and well-arranged, it's easier to find what you need, and the entire cooking process becomes more enjoyable. Here are some tips to help you organize your kitchen space for an anti-inflammatory lifestyle:

1. **Clear the Countertops**: Cluttered countertops can make your kitchen feel chaotic and uninviting. Keep only the essentials on the counters, such as a knife block, cutting boards, and perhaps a few frequently used appliances. Store everything else in cabinets or pantries.
2. **Organize Cabinets and Pantries**: Group similar items together in cabinets and pantries, making it easier to find what you need. Use clear containers or baskets to store items like grains, nuts, and seeds, and label them for easy identification.
3. **Create a Spice Drawer or Rack**: Spices are essential for adding flavor to anti-inflammatory dishes. Keep your spices organized in a drawer or rack, arranged alphabetically or by cuisine, for quick access.
4. **Designate a Produce Area**: Set aside a specific area in your refrigerator or on the counter for fresh produce. This will help you keep track of what you have and encourage you to use up perishable items before they spoil.
5. **Utilize Vertical Space**: Install shelves or hanging racks to make use of vertical space in your cabinets or pantry. This can help you

store items more efficiently and keep them within easy reach.
6. **Establish Zones**: Divide your kitchen into distinct zones for different tasks, such as food preparation, cooking, baking, and cleanup. This can streamline your workflow and make it easier to find the tools and ingredients you need for each task.
7. **Invest in Airtight Containers**: Store dry goods like grains, nuts, and seeds in airtight containers to keep them fresh and prevent pests or moisture from getting in.
8. **Label and Date**: Use labels and dates on containers and jars to keep track of when items were opened or purchased. This can help you rotate your stock and avoid waste.
9. **Purge and Declutter Regularly**: Go through your kitchen periodically and get rid of any expired, unused, or duplicate items. This will help keep your space organized and prevent clutter from accumulating.
10. **Make it Accessible**: Arrange your kitchen in a way that makes it easy for everyone in your household to access and use the space comfortably, regardless of their height or mobility.

Meal Planning and Preparation

Adopting an anti-inflammatory diet requires a bit of planning and preparation to ensure you have a variety of nutrient-dense, whole foods on hand. Meal planning can help you stay organized, save time, and reduce stress during the week. Here are some tips for effective meal planning and preparation:

1. **Create a Weekly Meal Plan**: Take some time each week to plan out your meals for the upcoming days. Consider your schedule, dietary preferences, and any leftovers you may have. Use a calendar or a dedicated meal planning app to help you stay organized.
2. **Make a Grocery List**: Once you have your meal plan in place, create a comprehensive grocery list. Check your pantry, refrigerator, and freezer to see what you already have, and then make a list of the items you need to purchase.
3. **Batch Cook and Prep**: Set aside some time on the weekends or your free days to batch cook and prepare ingredients for the week ahead. This could include cooking grains like quinoa or brown rice, roasting vegetables, marinating proteins, or making a big pot of soup or chili.

4. **Utilize Leftovers**: When planning your meals, consider how you can repurpose leftovers into new dishes. For example, leftover roasted vegetables can be used in a frittata or a grain bowl the next day.
5. **Invest in Meal Prep Containers**: Invest in high-quality, airtight containers to store prepped ingredients and meals. This will help keep your food fresh and make it easy to grab and go during busy weekdays.
6. **Plan for Variety**: To ensure you're getting a wide range of nutrients, plan for a variety of colors, textures, and flavors in your meals. Include a mix of fruits, vegetables, whole grains, lean proteins, and healthy fats.
7. **Consider Dietary Restrictions**: If you or someone in your household has specific dietary restrictions or allergies, plan your meals accordingly and ensure you have suitable alternatives available.
8. **Stay Flexible**: While meal planning is essential, allow for some flexibility in your schedule. Life can be unpredictable, and having a few easy-to-prepare options on hand can help you stay on track even when plans change.
9. **Involve Family Members**: If you're cooking for others, consider involving them in the meal planning process. This can help ensure everyone's preferences are taken into account

and encourage buy-in for the healthy meals you'll be preparing.
10. **Make It Enjoyable**: Meal planning and preparation shouldn't feel like a chore. Find ways to make it enjoyable, whether it's listening to music, trying new recipes, or involving your loved ones in the process.

Easy Recipes for Busy Mornings

Scrambled Eggs or Tofu with Spinach

Prep Time: 5 minutes
Cook Time: 10 minutes

Ingredients:
- 2 eggs or 1/2 package firm tofu, drained and crumbled
- 1 cup fresh baby spinach
- 1/2 bell pepper, diced
- 1/4 cup diced onion
- 1 clove garlic, minced
- 1 tsp olive oil or avocado oil
- 1/2 tsp ground turmeric

- Salt and pepper to taste

Instructions:
1. Heat oil in a skillet over medium heat.
2. Add onion and sauté for 2 minutes.
3. Add garlic and bell pepper, cook 1 minute.
4. Add spinach and turmeric, cook until spinach is wilted.
5. Push veggies to the side and scramble in eggs/tofu. Season with salt and pepper.

Nutritional Info (per serving, egg version):
Calories: 200, Protein: 13g, Fiber: 3g, Healthy Fats: 12g

Quinoa Breakfast Bowl

Prep Time: 5 minutes
Cook Time: 15 minutes

Ingredients:
- 1 cup cooked quinoa
- 1/2 cup fresh blueberries
- 2 tbsp sliced almonds
- 1 tbsp hemp seeds

- 1 tsp ground cinnamon
- Unsweetened almond milk for serving

Instructions:
1. In a saucepan, reheat the cooked quinoa over medium heat.
2. Transfer quinoa to a bowl and top with blueberries, almonds, hemp seeds, and cinnamon.
3. Drizzle with a splash of almond milk before serving.

Nutritional Info (per serving):
Calories: 340, Protein: 12g, Fiber: 9g, Healthy Fats: 16g

Breakfast Tacos

Prep Time: 10 minutes
Cook Time: 15 minutes

Ingredients:
- 4 whole grain tortillas or taco shells
- 1/2 cup black beans, rinsed and drained
- 1/2 cup diced bell peppers
- 1/4 cup diced onion

- 2 eggs, scrambled
- 1/4 cup salsa
- 1/4 avocado, sliced
- 2 tbsp chopped cilantro

Instructions:
1. In a skillet, sauté bell peppers and onions until softened.
2. Push veggies to the side and scramble in the eggs.
3. Warm the tortillas/taco shells.
4. Fill each with scrambled eggs, black beans, salsa, avocado, and cilantro.

Nutritional Info (per 2 tacos):
Calories: 380, Protein: 18g, Fiber: 15g, Healthy Fats: 13g

Green Smoothie with Kale

Prep Time: 5 minutes

Ingredients:
- 1 cup unsweetened almond milk
- 1 banana
- 1 cup packed kale leaves

- 1/2 cup frozen pineapple chunks
- 1 tbsp ground flaxseed
- 1 tsp grated ginger (optional)

Instructions:
1. Add all ingredients to a blender and blend until smooth.
2. Pour into a glass and enjoy!

Nutritional Info (per serving):
Calories: 250, Protein: 4g, Fiber: 7g, Healthy Fats: 5g

Buckwheat Pancakes

Prep Time: 10 minutes
Cook Time: 15 minutes

Ingredients:
- 1 cup buckwheat flour
- 1 tsp baking powder
- 1/2 tsp baking soda
- 1/4 tsp salt
- 1 cup unsweetened almond milk
- 1 tbsp apple cider vinegar

- 1 egg
- 1 tbsp maple syrup
- 1 tsp vanilla extract
- Coconut oil or avocado oil for cooking

Instructions:
1. In a bowl, whisk together the dry ingredients.
2. In another bowl, whisk the wet ingredients.
3. Pour the wet into the dry and mix just until combined.
4. Heat a non-stick skillet over medium heat and grease with oil.
5. Pour 1/4 cup batter per pancake and cook 2-3 minutes per side.
6. Serve warm with fresh berries, nut butter, or maple syrup.

Nutritional Info (makes 8 pancakes):
Calories: 140, Protein: 4g, Fiber: 4g, Healthy Fats: 3g (per 2 pancakes)

Veggie & Hummus Wrap

Prep Time: 10 minutes

Ingredients:
- 1 whole grain tortilla or flatbread
- 1/4 cup hummus
- 1/2 cup shredded carrots
- 1/4 cup chopped bell pepper
- 1/4 cup arugula or spinach
- 2 tbsp crumbled feta or goat cheese (optional)

Instructions:
1. Spread the hummus onto the tortilla/flatbread.
2. Layer with shredded carrots, bell pepper, greens, and cheese if using.
3. Roll up tightly and slice in half to serve.

Nutritional Info (per serving):
Calories: 330, Protein: 12g, Fiber: 9g, Healthy Fats: 11g

Quinoa Bowl with Dried Apricots

Prep Time: 5 minutes
Cook Time: 15 minutes

Ingredients:
- 1 cup cooked quinoa

- 1/4 cup dried apricots, chopped
- 2 tbsp sliced almonds
- 1 tbsp chia seeds
- 1/2 tsp ground cinnamon
- Unsweetened almond milk for serving

Instructions:
1. In a saucepan, reheat the cooked quinoa over medium heat.
2. Transfer to a bowl and top with chopped apricots, almonds, chia, and cinnamon.
3. Drizzle with a splash of almond milk before serving.

Nutritional Info (per serving):
Calories: 360, Protein: 10g, Fiber: 9g, Healthy Fats: 13g

Cottage Cheese or Dairy-Free Yogurt Bowl

Prep Time: 5 minutes

Ingredients:

- 1 cup low-fat cottage cheese or unsweetened dairy-free yogurt
- 1/2 cup fresh or frozen berries
- 2 tbsp sliced almonds or chopped walnuts
- 1 tbsp ground flaxseed
- 1 tsp honey or maple syrup (optional)

Instructions:
1. In a bowl, place the cottage cheese or yogurt.
2. Top with berries, nuts, flaxseed, and a drizzle of honey/maple syrup if desired.
3. Can also add a sprinkle of cinnamon or vanilla extract.

Nutritional Info (per serving, cottage cheese version):
Calories: 290, Protein: 28g, Fiber: 4g, Healthy Fats: 13g

Breakfast Burrito

Prep Time: 10 minutes
Cook Time: 10 minutes

Ingredients:

- 2 eggs, scrambled
- 1 whole wheat tortilla
- 1/4 cup black beans, rinsed and drained
- 1/4 avocado, diced
- 2 tbsp salsa
- 1 tbsp chopped cilantro

Instructions:
1. Scramble the eggs in a skillet.
2. Warm the tortilla.
3. Layer the scrambled eggs, black beans, avocado, salsa, and cilantro.
4. Roll up tightly into a burrito.

Nutritional Info (per burrito):
Calories: 400, Protein: 19g, Fiber: 11g, Healthy Fats: 17g

Oatmeal Bowl with Poached Egg

Prep Time: 5 minutes
Cook Time: 10 minutes

Ingredients:
- 1 cup cooked steel-cut or rolled oats

- 1 poached egg
- 1/4 avocado, sliced
- 1 tbsp pepitas (pumpkin seeds)
- Hot sauce or red pepper flakes for serving

Instructions:
1. Prepare oats according to package directions.
2. Poach the egg while oats are cooking.
3. Scoop oats into a bowl, top with poached egg, avocado, and pepitas.
4. Add a dash of hot sauce or red pepper flakes if desired.

Nutritional Info (per serving):
Calories: 410, Protein: 17g, Fiber: 14g, Healthy Fats: 19g

Whole Grain Waffles

Prep Time: 10 minutes
Cook Time: 15 minutes

Ingredients:
- 1 cup whole wheat or oat flour

- 1 tsp baking powder
- 1/4 tsp salt
- 1 egg
- 3/4 cup unsweetened almond milk
- 2 tbsp avocado or melted coconut oil
- 1 tsp vanilla extract
- Toppings: fresh berries, pure maple syrup, nut butter

Instructions:
1. In a bowl, whisk together the flour, baking powder and salt.
2. In another bowl, whisk the egg, then add milk, oil and vanilla.
3. Pour the wet into the dry and whisk until just combined.
4. Pour batter onto a preheated waffle iron and cook per manufacturer's instructions.
5. Serve warm with desired toppings.

Nutritional Info (makes 4 waffles):
Calories: 220, Protein: 6g, Fiber: 4g, Healthy Fats: 11g (per waffle)

Veggie & Tofu Scramble

Prep Time: 10 minutes
Cook Time: 10 minutes

Ingredients:
- 1/2 block firm tofu, pressed and crumbled
- 1 cup sliced mushrooms
- 1 cup baby spinach
- 1/2 bell pepper, diced
- 1 clove garlic, minced
- 1 tbsp olive or avocado oil
- 1 tsp ground turmeric
- Salt and pepper to taste

Instructions:
1. Heat oil in a skillet over medium heat.
2. Add garlic and sauté for 1 minute.
3. Add mushrooms and bell pepper, sauté 2-3 minutes.
4. Add crumbled tofu and turmeric, toss to coat.
5. Add spinach and cook until wilted. Season with salt and pepper.

Nutritional Info (per serving):

Calories: 170, Protein: 13g, Fiber: 4g, Healthy Fats: 10g

Breakfast Muffins Combo

Prep Time: 15 minutes
Cook Time: 20 minutes

Ingredients:
- 1 cup oat flour
- 1 tsp baking powder
- 1/2 tsp baking soda
- 1/2 tsp cinnamon
- 1 ripe banana, mashed
- 1/2 cup unsweetened applesauce
- 1/4 cup unsweetened almond milk
- 2 eggs
- 1/4 cup blueberries or chopped walnuts (optional)

Instructions:
1. Preheat oven to 375°F and grease a muffin tin.
2. In a bowl, mix the dry ingredients.
3. In another bowl, mix the wet ingredients.
4. Pour the wet into the dry and fold in berries/nuts if using.

5. Divide batter into muffin cups.
6. Bake 18-20 minutes until a toothpick comes out clean.

Nutritional Info (makes 10 muffins):
Calories: 100, Protein: 3g, Fiber: 2g, Healthy Fats: 2g (per muffin)

Smoked Salmon & Cream Cheese

Prep Time: 5 minutes

Ingredients:
- 2 slices whole grain bread, toasted
- 2 oz smoked salmon
- 2 tbsp cream cheese or dairy-free cream cheese
- 1 tbsp capers
- 1 tsp lemon zest
- Fresh dill for garnish

Instructions:
1. Lightly toast the bread
2. Spread each slice with 1 tbsp cream cheese
3. Top with smoked salmon, capers and lemon zest
4. Garnish with fresh dill

Nutritional Info (per serving):
Calories: 250, Protein: 18g, Fiber: 4g, Healthy Fats: 9g

Tropical Smoothie Bowl

Prep Time: 5 minutes
Cook Time: None

Ingredients:
- 1 frozen banana
- 1 cup frozen mango chunks
- 1/2 cup unsweetened coconut milk
- 1/4 cup plain Greek yogurt
- 1 tbsp chia seeds or ground flaxseeds
- Toppings: shredded coconut, sliced kiwi, granola

Instructions:
1. Add banana, mango, coconut milk, yogurt, and chia/flax seeds to a blender.
2. Blend until smooth and thick.
3. Pour into a bowl and top with shredded coconut, kiwi slices, and granola.

Nutritional Value (per serving):

Calories: 320, Protein: 8g, Carbs: 55g, Fiber: 8g, Fat: 9g

Turkey Bacon Avocado Wrap

Prep Time: 10 minutes
Cook Time: 5 minutes

Ingredients:
- 2 slices whole wheat tortilla or wrap
- 2 slices turkey bacon, cooked
- 1/4 avocado, mashed
- 1 egg, scrambled
- 1/4 cup baby spinach
- 1 tbsp salsa

Instructions:
1. Cook turkey bacon according to package instructions.
2. Scramble the egg in a small non-stick skillet.
3. Lay the tortilla flat and spread mashed avocado down the center.
4. Top with scrambled egg, turkey bacon, spinach, and salsa.

5. Wrap up tightly and enjoy!

Nutritional Value (per serving):
Calories: 330, Protein: 18g, Carbs: 28g, Fiber: 7g, Fat: 17g

Vegetable Frittata

Prep Time: 10 minutes
Cook Time: 20 minutes

Ingredients:
- 6 eggs
- 1/4 cup milk
- 1 cup mixed vegetables (bell peppers, onions, mushrooms, spinach)
- 2 tbsp shredded cheese
- Salt and pepper to taste

Instructions:
1. Preheat oven to 375°F (190°C).
2. In a bowl, whisk together eggs and milk. Season with salt and pepper.

3. In an oven-safe skillet, sauté mixed vegetables until tender.
4. Pour egg mixture over vegetables and sprinkle with shredded cheese.
5. Bake for 15-20 minutes until frittata is set in the middle.
6. Slice and serve warm.

Nutritional Value (per serving):
Calories: 210, Protein: 16g, Carbs: 6g, Fiber: 2g, Fat: 13g

Tuna Salad Wrap

Prep Time: 10 minutes
Cook Time: None

Ingredients:
- 1 (5 oz) can tuna, drained
- 2 tbsp plain Greek yogurt
- 1 tbsp diced celery
- 1 tbsp diced red onion
- 1 tsp Dijon mustard

- Salt and pepper to taste
- 1 whole wheat tortilla or wrap
- Mixed greens or spinach

Instructions:
1. In a bowl, mix together tuna, yogurt, celery, onion, mustard, salt, and pepper.
2. Lay the tortilla flat and place mixed greens down the center.
3. Top with tuna salad mixture.
4. Wrap up tightly and enjoy!

Nutritional Value (per serving):
Calories: 280, Protein: 28g, Carbs: 25g, Fiber: 5g, Fat: 7g

Blueberry Almond Overnight Oats

Prep Time: 5 minutes (plus overnight soaking)
Cook Time: None

Ingredients:
- 1/2 cup rolled oats
- 1/2 cup unsweetened almond milk
- 1/4 cup Greek yogurt

- 1 tbsp maple syrup
- 1/2 tsp vanilla extract
- 1/2 cup blueberries
- 2 tbsp sliced almonds

Instructions:
1. In a jar or bowl, combine oats, almond milk, yogurt, maple syrup, and vanilla. Mix well.
2. Gently fold in blueberries.
3. Cover and refrigerate overnight.
4. Top with sliced almonds before serving.

Nutritional Value (per serving):
Calories: 325, Protein: 11g, Carbs: 46g, Fiber: 7g, Fat: 11g

Peanut Butter Banana Smoothie Bowl

Prep Time: 5 minutes
Cook Time: None

Ingredients:
- 1 banana
- 1/2 cup milk of choice

- 2 tbsp peanut butter
- 1 tsp honey
- 1/2 cup ice cubes
- Toppings: granola, sliced banana, cinnamon

Instructions:
1. Add banana, milk, peanut butter, honey, and ice to a blender. Blend until smooth.
2. Pour into a bowl and top with granola, sliced banana, and a sprinkle of cinnamon.

Nutritional Value (per serving):
Calories: 370, Protein: 13g, Carbs: 53g, Fiber: 6g, Fat: 16g

Egg and Veggie Wrap

Prep Time: 5 minutes
Cook Time: 5 minutes

Ingredients:
- 1 whole wheat tortilla or wrap
- 1 egg, scrambled

- 1/4 cup sautéed vegetables (spinach, bell peppers, onions)
- 2 tbsp shredded cheese

Instructions:
1. Scramble the egg in a small non-stick skillet.
2. Sauté vegetables until tender.
3. Lay tortilla flat and layer scrambled egg, sautéed veggies, and shredded cheese.
4. Roll up tightly and enjoy!

Nutritional Value (per serving):
Calories: 290, Protein: 16g, Carbs: 26g, Fiber: 4g, Fat: 13g

Spinach and Feta Egg Muffins

Prep Time: 10 minutes
Cook Time: 20 minutes

Ingredients:
- 6 eggs
- 1/4 cup milk
- 1 cup fresh spinach, chopped

- 1/4 cup crumbled feta cheese
- Salt and pepper to taste

Instructions:
1. Preheat oven to 375°F (190°C). Grease a muffin tin.
2. In a bowl, whisk together eggs and milk. Season with salt and pepper.
3. Stir in spinach and feta cheese.
4. Pour mixture evenly into muffin cups.
5. Bake for 18-20 minutes until set.
6. Let cool slightly before removing from tin.

Nutritional Value (per muffin):
Calories: 90, Protein: 7g, Carbs: 1g, Fiber: 0g, Fat: 6g

Bacon and Cheddar Egg Muffins

Prep Time: 15 minutes
Cook Time: 20 minutes

Ingredients:
- 6 eggs

- 1/4 cup milk
- 4 slices bacon, cooked and crumbled
- 1/2 cup shredded cheddar cheese
- 2 green onions, sliced
- Salt and pepper to taste

Instructions:
1. Preheat oven to 375°F (190°C). Grease a muffin tin.
2. In a bowl, whisk together eggs and milk. Season with salt and pepper.
3. Stir in bacon, cheddar cheese, and green onions.
4. Pour mixture evenly into muffin cups.
5. Bake for 18-20 minutes until set.

Nutritional Value (per muffin):
Calories: 140, Protein: 9g, Carbs: 1g, Fiber: 0g, Fat: 11g

With this variety of quick and easy anti-inflammatory breakfast recipes, you can start your day off on the right foot with nutrient-dense ingredients like whole grains, fruits, veggies, proteins and healthy fats. Mix and match to keep things interesting!

Breakfast Ideas for Meal Preparation

Here are some make-ahead anti-inflammatory breakfast ideas perfect for meal prep, including prep/cook times, ingredients, instructions, and nutritional information:

Egg Muffin Cups

Prep Time: 10 minutes
Cook Time: 20 minutes

Ingredients:
- 8 eggs
- 1/4 cup milk (dairy or plant-based)
- 1 cup chopped veggies like bell peppers, onions, spinach
- 1/2 cup shredded cheese (omit for dairy-free)
- Salt and pepper to taste
- Optional add-ins: turkey bacon, ham, etc.

Instructions:
1. Preheat oven to 350°F. Grease a 12-cup muffin tin.

2. In a bowl, whisk together eggs and milk. Season with salt and pepper.
3. Stir in chopped veggies, cheese if using, and any other add-ins.
4. Pour egg mixture evenly into prepared muffin cups.
5. Bake for 16-20 minutes until centers are set.
6. Allow to cool slightly before removing from tin. Refrigerate for make-ahead breakfasts.

Nutritional Info (makes 12 cups):
Calories: 80, Protein: 6g, Healthy Fats: 5g (per egg cup, without add-ins)

Smoothie Packs

Prep Time: 10 minutes

Ingredients (Makes 5 Smoothie Packs):
- 2 ripe bananas, sliced and frozen
- 2 cups fresh spinach
- 1 cup frozen mixed berries
- 1/2 cup plain Greek yogurt (or dairy-free yogurt)
- 1/4 cup old-fashioned oats
- 2 tbsp nut or seed butter

Instructions:
1. Distribute all ingredients evenly between 5 quart-sized freezer bags.
2. Seal bags, squeezing out any excess air.
3. Freeze for up to 3 months.
4. To blend, add 1 cup milk or juice to the bag contents and blend until smooth.

Nutritional Info (per smoothie pack):
Calories: 235, Protein: 10g, Fiber: 6g, Healthy Fats: 8g

Coconut Yogurt Parfait

Prep Time: 10 minutes

Ingredients (Makes 4 parfaits):
- 2 cups unsweetened coconut yogurt
- 1 cup fresh or frozen mixed berries
- 1/2 cup granola (low sugar/no added oils)
- 2 tbsp chia seeds
- 1 tsp vanilla extract
- 1/4 tsp ground cinnamon

Instructions:
1. In 4 mason jars or portable containers, layer 1/4 cup yogurt, 1/4 cup berries, 2 tbsp granola, and 1/2 tsp chia seeds.
2. Repeat layers ending with berries and granola on top.
3. Drizzle with vanilla and sprinkle with cinnamon.
4. Seal containers and refrigerate up to 5 days.

Nutrition (per parfait):
Calories: 205, Protein: 6g, Fiber: 6g, Healthy Fats: 10g

Breakfast Muffins

Prep Time: 15 minutes
Cook Time: 18 minutes

Ingredients (Makes 12 muffins):
- 1 1/2 cups oat flour
- 1 tsp baking powder
- 1/2 tsp baking soda
- 1/2 tsp cinnamon
- 1/4 tsp salt
- 1 cup mashed ripe banana (about 2 large)

- 1/2 cup unsweetened applesauce
- 1/4 cup maple syrup
- 2 eggs
- 1 tsp vanilla
- 1/2 cup fresh or frozen blueberries (optional)

Instructions:
1. Preheat oven to 350°F and grease a 12-cup muffin tin.
2. In a bowl, whisk together the dry ingredients.
3. In another bowl, mix together the wet ingredients.
4. Pour the wet into the dry and fold just until combined. Gently fold in blueberries if using.
5. Divide batter evenly into prepared muffin cups.
6. Bake 16-18 minutes until a toothpick inserted in the center comes out clean.
7. Cool completely before storing in an airtight container up to 5 days.

Nutrition (per muffin):
Calories: 120, Protein: 3g, Fiber: 2g, Healthy Fats: 2g

Breakfast Burrito Wraps

Prep Time: 20 minutes
Cook Time: 15 minutes

Ingredients (Makes 6 wraps):
- 6 whole wheat tortillas
- 6 eggs, scrambled
- 1 cup diced bell pepper
- 1/2 cup diced onion
- 1 cup black beans, rinsed and drained
- 1 avocado, diced
- 1/2 cup salsa
- 1/2 cup shredded cheese (optional)

Instructions:
1. Scramble the eggs in a skillet over medium heat.
2. In the same skillet, sauté the bell pepper and onion for 2-3 minutes.
3. Allow the egg mixture and veggies to cool slightly.
4. Lay the tortillas out and layer each with scrambled eggs, sauteed veggies, black beans, avocado, salsa, and cheese if using.
5. Roll up tightly into burritos and wrap individually in foil or parchment paper.

6. Refrigerate up to 5 days. Reheat in microwave or oven before eating.

Nutrition (per burrito):
Calories: 300, Protein: 15g, Fiber: 10g, Healthy Fats: 13g

Steel-Cut Oats with Almond Butter

Prep Time: 5 minutes
Cook Time: 25 minutes

Ingredients (Serves 4):
- 1 cup steel-cut oats
- 4 cups unsweetened almond milk
- 1 tsp cinnamon
- 1/4 tsp nutmeg
- 1 tbsp chia seeds
- 1/4 cup almond butter
- 1 cup fresh or frozen mixed berries

Instructions:
1. In a saucepan, combine the oats, milk, cinnamon, nutmeg and chia seeds.

2. Bring to a boil, then reduce heat and simmer for 20-25 minutes, stirring frequently, until oats are thick and creamy.
3. Remove from heat and stir in the almond butter until combined.
4. Divide oatmeal into 4 containers and top each with 1/4 cup berries.
5. Seal and refrigerate up to 5 days. Reheat with a splash of milk if desired.

Nutrition (per serving):
Calories: 305, Protein: 8g, Fiber: 8g, Healthy Fats: 16g

Protein-Packed Quinoa Bowl

Prep Time: 10 minutes
Cook Time: 20 minutes

Ingredients (Makes 4 servings):
- 1 cup uncooked quinoa
- 1 cup shredded chicken or cooked lentils
- 1 cup cherry tomatoes, halved
- 1 avocado, diced
- 1/4 cup chopped green onions

- 2 tbsp pepitas (pumpkin seeds)
- 2 tbsp olive oil
- 2 tbsp lemon juice
- Salt and pepper to taste

Instructions:
1. Cook the quinoa according to package instructions. Allow to cool slightly.
2. In a large bowl, mix together the cooked quinoa, shredded chicken/lentils, tomatoes, avocado, and green onions.
3. Drizzle with olive oil and lemon juice. Season with salt and pepper to taste.
4. Portion into 4 containers and top each with 1/2 tbsp pepitas.
5. Refrigerate up to 4 days.

Nutrition (per serving):
Calories: 370, Protein: 19g, Fiber: 9g, Healthy Fats: 18g

Baked Oatmeal Squares

Prep Time: 10 minutes
Cook Time: 30 minutes

Ingredients (Makes 9 squares):
- 2 cups rolled oats
- 1 tsp baking powder
- 1 tsp cinnamon
- 1/4 tsp salt
- 1 cup unsweetened almond milk
- 1 egg
- 1/4 cup mashed ripe banana
- 1/4 cup applesauce
- 1 tsp vanilla extract
- 1/2 cup fresh or frozen blueberries

Instructions:
1. Preheat oven to 375°F. Grease an 8x8 inch baking pan.
2. In a bowl, mix together the oats, baking powder, cinnamon and salt.
3. In another bowl, whisk together the milk, egg, banana, applesauce and vanilla.
4. Pour the wet ingredients into the dry and mix until well combined.
5. Gently fold in the blueberries.
6. Pour into prepared pan and bake for 28-32 minutes until set.

7. Allow to cool completely before slicing into 9 squares.

Nutrition (per square):
Calories: 130, Protein: 4g, Fiber: 4g, Healthy Fats: 3g

Avocado and Smoked Salmon Toast

Prep Time: 10 minutes
Cook Time: 5 minutes (for eggs)

Ingredients (Makes 2 servings):
- 2 slices whole grain bread
- 1 avocado, mashed
- 4 oz smoked salmon
- 2 eggs, cooked to your liking
- 1 tsp everything bagel seasoning
- Lemon wedges for serving

Instructions:
1. Toast the bread and mash the avocado with a fork.
2. Spread the mashed avocado evenly over the toasted bread slices.
3. Cook the eggs to your desired doneness.

4. Top each avocado toast with 2 oz smoked salmon and 1 cooked egg.
5. Sprinkle with everything bagel seasoning.
6. Serve with lemon wedges for squeezing over top.

Nutrition (per serving):
Calories: 350, Protein: 20g, Fiber: 9g, Healthy Fats: 20g

Tofu Scramble Wraps

Prep Time: 10 minutes
Cook Time: 10 minutes

Ingredients (Makes 4 wraps):
- 1 tbsp olive oil
- 1/2 onion, diced
- 1 bell pepper, diced
- 1 package firm tofu, drained and crumbled
- 1 tsp turmeric
- 1 tsp garlic powder
- 1 tsp cumin
- Salt and pepper to taste
- 4 whole wheat tortillas
- 1/4 cup salsa per wrap

Instructions:
1. Heat oil in a skillet over medium heat. Cook onion for 2 minutes.
2. Add bell pepper and cook 3 more minutes until softened.
3. Crumble in the tofu and add spices. Cook 3-4 minutes until heated through.
4. Divide tofu scramble evenly among tortillas. Top each with 1/4 cup salsa.
5. Roll up tortillas and wrap individually. Refrigerate for up to 5 days.

Nutrition (per wrap):
Calories: 280, Protein: 15g, Fiber: 8g, Healthy Fats: 11g

Berry and Spinach Breakfast Smoothie Packs

Prep Time: 10 minutes

Ingredients (Makes 5 packs):
- 2 cups fresh spinach
- 2 cups frozen mixed berries
- 1 banana, sliced and frozen

- 1/2 cup plain Greek yogurt
- 2 tbsp ground flaxseed
- 1 tbsp almond butter

Instructions:
1. Divide all ingredients evenly between 5 quart-sized ziplock bags.
2. Seal bags, squeezing out excess air. Freeze for up to 3 months.
3. To blend, remove a bag from freezer and let thaw slightly.
4. Pour contents into a blender with 1 cup unsweetened plant milk and blend until smooth.

Nutrition (per smoothie pack):
Calories: 190, Protein: 9g, Fiber: 7g, Healthy Fats: 8g

Bircher Muesli

Prep Time: 10 minutes (plus overnight soaking)

Ingredients (Serves 4):
- 1 cup rolled oats
- 1 cup unsweetened plant-based milk

- 1/4 cup plain Greek yogurt
- 1 apple, grated
- 1 tbsp chia seeds
- 1 tsp cinnamon
- 1/4 cup chopped toasted nuts
- 1/4 cup fresh or frozen berries

Instructions:

1. In a bowl, combine oats, milk, yogurt, apple, chia seeds and cinnamon. Cover and refrigerate overnight.
2. In the morning, stir in chopped nuts and divide into 4 containers.
3. Top each serving with 1/4 cup berries.
4. Will keep refrigerated for up to 4 days.

Nutrition (per serving):
Calories: 245, Protein: 8g, Fiber: 8g, Healthy Fats: 9g

Fluffy Whole Wheat Pancakes

Prep Time: 10 minutes

Cook Time: 15 minutes

Makes: 8 pancakes

Ingredients:

- 1 cup whole wheat flour

- 2 tsp baking powder

- 1/2 tsp salt

- 1 tbsp sugar

- 1 egg

- 1 cup milk

- 2 tbsp melted butter or oil

- 1 tsp vanilla extract

Instructions:

1. In a large bowl, whisk together the flour, baking powder, salt, and sugar.

2. In a separate bowl, beat the egg, then whisk in the milk, melted butter, and vanilla.

3. Pour the wet ingredients into the dry ingredients and stir just until combined (do not overmix).

4. Heat a non-stick skillet or griddle over medium heat and grease lightly.

5. Pour 1/4 cup of batter onto the skillet for each pancake.

6. Cook until bubbles appear on the surface, then flip and cook until golden brown on both sides.

7. Serve warm with desired toppings like fresh fruits, maple syrup, or nut butter.

Nutritional Value (per pancake):

Calories: 135, Protein: 5g, Carbs: 18g, Fiber: 3g, Fat: 5g

Denver Omelet

Prep Time: 10 minutes

Cook Time: 10 minutes

Serves: 1

Ingredients:

- 3 eggs

- 1 tbsp butter

- 1/4 cup diced ham

- 1/4 cup diced bell pepper

- 1/4 cup diced onion

- 2 tbsp shredded cheddar cheese

- Salt and pepper to taste

Instructions:

1. Crack the eggs into a bowl and beat them with a fork. Season with salt and pepper.

2. Melt the butter in a non-stick skillet over medium heat.

3. Pour in the beaten eggs and let them sit for 20-30 seconds to set the bottom.

4. Using a spatula, gently push the cooked eggs towards the center, tilting the pan to allow the uncooked eggs to flow to the edges.

5. When the eggs are mostly set but still look moist, add the ham, bell pepper, and onion to one half of the omelet.

6. Sprinkle the cheddar cheese over the fillings.

7. Use the spatula to fold the other half of the omelet over the fillings.

8. Slide the omelet onto a plate and serve hot.

Nutritional Value (per serving):

Calories: 400, Protein: 25g, Carbs: 6g, Fiber: 1g, Fat: 28g

Quinoa Breakfast Bowl

Prep Time: 5 minutes

Cook Time: 20 minutes

Serves: 2

Ingredients:

- 1 cup cooked quinoa

- 1 cup unsweetened almond milk

- 1/2 cup mixed berries

- 2 tbsp sliced almonds

- 1 tbsp honey or maple syrup

- Pinch of cinnamon

Instructions:

1. In a saucepan, combine the cooked quinoa and almond milk. Heat over medium, stirring occasionally, until hot and slightly thickened.

2. Remove from heat and stir in the mixed berries, sliced almonds, honey/maple syrup, and cinnamon.

3. Divide between two bowls and serve warm.

Nutritional Value (per serving):

Calories: 320, Protein: 9g, Carbs: 52g, Fiber: 6g, Fat: 10g

Chorizo and Egg Breakfast Burrito

Prep Time: 10 minutes

Cook Time: 15 minutes

Serves: 2

Ingredients:

- 4 eggs

- 1/4 cup milk

- 1/2 cup cooked chorizo

- 1/4 cup diced bell pepper

- 1/4 cup diced onion

- 2 large whole wheat tortillas

- 1/4 cup shredded cheddar cheese

- Salt and pepper to taste

Instructions:

1. In a bowl, whisk together the eggs and milk. Season with salt and pepper.

2. In a non-stick skillet, cook the egg mixture over medium heat, stirring occasionally, until scrambled.

3. In the same skillet, sauté the chorizo, bell pepper, and onion until the vegetables are tender.

4. Warm the tortillas according to package instructions.

5. Divide the scrambled eggs, chorizo mixture, and shredded cheese between the two tortillas.

6. Fold the sides inward and roll up tightly into burritos.

7. Serve warm with salsa or hot sauce on the side.

Nutritional Value (per burrito):

Calories: 550, Protein: 30g, Carbs: 42g, Fiber: 7g, Fat: 28g

Savory Cheddar Chive Waffles

Prep Time: 10 minutes

Cook Time: 20 minutes

Makes: 6 waffles

Ingredients:

- 1 1/2 cups all-purpose flour

- 2 tsp baking powder

- 1 tsp salt

- 1/4 tsp black pepper

- 2 eggs

- 1 1/4 cups milk

- 1/4 cup melted butter or oil

- 1 cup shredded cheddar cheese

- 1/4 cup chopped fresh chives

Instructions:

1. In a large bowl, whisk together the flour, baking powder, salt, and black pepper.

2. In a separate bowl, beat the eggs, then whisk in the milk and melted butter.

3. Pour the wet ingredients into the dry ingredients and stir just until combined (do not overmix).

4. Gently fold in the shredded cheddar and chopped chives.

5. Preheat your waffle iron and grease it lightly.

6. Pour batter onto the hot waffle iron, using about 1/2 cup per waffle.

7. Cook until golden brown and crispy.

8. Serve warm with your favorite toppings like avocado, salsa, or fried eggs.

Nutritional Value (per waffle):

Calories: 320, Protein: 11g, Carbs: 30g, Fiber: 1g, Fat: 18g

Vegetarian and Vegan Options

Here is the "Vegetarian and Vegan Options" section with recipes including prep/cook times, ingredients, instructions and nutritional information:

Lentil and Walnut Meatballs

Prep Time: 20 minutes
Cook Time: 30 minutes
Servings: 4

Ingredients:
- 1 cup cooked green lentils
- 1 cup walnuts
- 1 flax egg (1 tbsp ground flaxseed + 3 tbsp water)
- 1/2 cup breadcrumbs
- 1/4 cup grated vegan parmesan
- 1 clove garlic, minced
- 1 tsp Italian seasoning
- Salt and pepper to taste

Instructions:
1. Preheat oven to 375°F (190°C). Line a baking sheet with parchment paper.
2. Pulse walnuts in a food processor until crumbly. Add lentils, flax egg, breadcrumbs, vegan parmesan, garlic, Italian seasoning, salt, and pepper. Pulse until well combined but still slightly chunky.
3. Roll mixture into 1-inch balls and place on the prepared baking sheet.

4. Bake for 25-30 minutes, turning halfway, until golden brown and firm.
5. Serve with marinara sauce or desired dipping sauce.

Nutritional Value (per serving, about 4 meatballs): Calories: 280, Protein: 12g, Carbs: 24g, Fiber: 7g, Fat: 16g

Mediterranean Quinoa Bowl

Prep Time: 15 minutes
Cook Time: 20 minutes
Servings: 2

Ingredients:
- 1 cup quinoa, rinsed
- 2 cups vegetable broth
- 1 cup diced cucumber
- 1 cup cherry tomatoes, halved
- 1/2 cup pitted Kalamata olives
- 1/4 cup crumbled feta or vegan feta
- 2 tbsp chopped fresh parsley
- Lemon wedges for serving

Dressing:
- 2 tbsp olive oil
- 1 tbsp lemon juice
- 1 tsp Dijon mustard
- Salt and pepper to taste

Instructions:
1. In a saucepan, bring quinoa and vegetable broth to a boil. Reduce heat, cover, and simmer for 15-18 minutes until liquid is absorbed.
2. In a small bowl, whisk together the dressing ingredients.
3. In a large bowl, combine cooked quinoa, cucumber, tomatoes, olives, feta, and parsley.
4. Drizzle the dressing over the quinoa mixture and toss to coat.
5. Serve with lemon wedges.

Nutritional Value (per serving):
Calories: 480, Protein: 14g, Carbs: 54g, Fiber: 8g, Fat: 23g

Kale and Roasted Vegetable Salad

Prep Time: 15 minutes
Cook Time: 30 minutes
Servings: 4

Ingredients:
- 1 bunch kale, stemmed and chopped
- 1 large sweet potato, diced
- 1 red bell pepper, diced
- 1 red onion, diced
- 2 tbsp olive oil
- Salt and pepper to taste
- 1/4 cup toasted pumpkin seeds
- 1/4 cup crumbled feta or vegan feta (optional)

Dressing:
- 2 tbsp olive oil
- 2 tbsp apple cider vinegar
- 1 tsp Dijon mustard
- 1 tsp maple syrup

Instructions:
1. Preheat oven to 400°F (200°C). Line a baking sheet with parchment paper.

2. Toss sweet potato, bell pepper, and onion with 2 tbsp olive oil, salt, and pepper. Spread on the prepared baking sheet.
3. Roast for 25-30 minutes, tossing halfway, until tender and lightly browned.
4. In a small bowl, whisk together the dressing ingredients.
5. In a large bowl, combine the chopped kale and roasted vegetables. Drizzle with the dressing and toss to coat.
6. Top with toasted pumpkin seeds and feta or vegan feta, if desired.

Nutritional Value (per serving):
Calories: 260, Protein: 5g, Carbs: 28g, Fiber: 5g, Fat: 16g

Vegetable Soup

Prep Time: 15 minutes
Cook Time: 30 minutes
Servings: 4

Ingredients:

- 1 tbsp olive oil
- 1 onion, diced
- 2 carrots, sliced
- 2 celery stalks, sliced
- 2 cloves garlic, minced
- 4 cups vegetable broth
- 1 (14.5 oz) can diced tomatoes
- 1 cup green beans, cut into 1-inch pieces
- 1 cup diced zucchini
- 1 tsp dried basil
- Salt and pepper to taste
- 2 cups baby spinach or kale

Instructions:
1. In a large pot, heat olive oil over medium heat. Add onion, carrots, and celery. Cook for 5 minutes until softened.
2. Add garlic and cook for 1 minute until fragrant.
3. Pour in vegetable broth, diced tomatoes, green beans, zucchini, basil, salt, and pepper.
4. Bring to a boil, then reduce heat and simmer for 15-20 minutes until vegetables are tender.
5. Stir in spinach or kale and cook for 2-3 minutes until wilted.
6. Adjust seasoning with salt and pepper if needed.
7. Serve hot.

Nutritional Value (per serving):
Calories: 120, Protein: 4g, Carbs: 19g, Fiber: 6g, Fat: 4g

Chickpea Curry

Prep Time: 10 minutes
Cook Time: 25 minutes
Servings: 4

Ingredients:
- 1 tbsp olive oil
- 1 onion, diced
- 3 cloves garlic, minced
- 1 tbsp grated fresh ginger
- 1 tbsp curry powder
- 1 tsp garam masala
- 1 tsp ground cumin
- 1/2 tsp cayenne pepper (optional)
- 1 (14.5 oz) can diced tomatoes
- 1 (14 oz) can chickpeas, drained and rinsed
- 1 cup vegetable broth
- 1/2 cup coconut milk

- Salt and pepper to taste
- Chopped fresh cilantro for garnish

Instructions:
1. In a large skillet or pot, heat olive oil over medium heat. Add onion and cook for 5 minutes until softened.
2. Add garlic, ginger, curry powder, garam masala, cumin, and cayenne (if using). Cook for 1 minute until fragrant.
3. Stir in diced tomatoes, chickpeas, vegetable broth, and coconut milk. Season with salt and pepper.
4. Bring to a simmer and cook for 15-20 minutes, stirring occasionally, until thickened.
5. Taste and adjust seasoning if needed.
6. Garnish with fresh cilantro and serve over basmati rice or with naan bread.

Nutritional Value (per serving):
Calories: 300, Protein: 10g, Carbs: 40g, Fiber: 9g, Fat: 13g

Chickpea Salad

Prep Time: 10 minutes

Chill Time: 30 minutes
Serves: 4

Ingredients:
- 1 (15 oz) can chickpeas, drained and rinsed
- 1 celery stalk, diced
- 1/4 cup diced red onion
- 2 tablespoons chopped parsley
- 2 tablespoons vegan mayonnaise
- 1 tablespoon Dijon mustard
- 1 tablespoon lemon juice
- Salt and pepper to taste

Instructions:
1. In a medium bowl, mash the chickpeas lightly with a fork or potato masher, leaving some chickpeas whole.
2. Add the celery, red onion, and parsley, and stir to combine.
3. In a small bowl, whisk together the vegan mayonnaise, Dijon mustard, and lemon juice.
4. Pour the dressing over the chickpea mixture and stir to coat evenly.
5. Season with salt and pepper to taste.
6. Chill for at least 30 minutes before serving to allow flavors to meld.

Nutritional Information (per serving):
Calories: 160
Protein: 6g
Carbs: 21g
Fiber: 6g
Fat: 5g

Roasted Vegetable Buddha Bowl

Prep Time: 15 minutes
Cook Time: 30 minutes
Serves: 4

Ingredients:
- 1 sweet potato, cubed
- 1 cup brussels sprouts, halved
- 1 cup cauliflower florets
- 2 tablespoons olive oil
- 1 teaspoon smoked paprika
- Salt and pepper to taste
- 1 cup cooked quinoa
- 1 avocado, sliced
- 1/4 cup roasted chickpeas

- 2 tablespoons tahini dressing

Instructions:
1. Preheat oven to 400°F (200°C).
2. On a baking sheet, toss the sweet potato, brussels sprouts, and cauliflower with olive oil, smoked paprika, salt, and pepper.
3. Roast for 25-30 minutes, or until vegetables are tender and lightly browned.
4. Divide the cooked quinoa among 4 bowls.
5. Top each bowl with the roasted vegetables, sliced avocado, and roasted chickpeas.
6. Drizzle with tahini dressing.

Nutritional Information (per serving):
Calories: 330
Protein: 9g
Carbs: 39g
Fiber: 11g
Fat: 17g

Lentil Soup

Prep Time: 10 minutes
Cook Time: 40 minutes
Serves: 6

Ingredients:
- 1 cup dried green lentils
- 1 onion, diced
- 2 carrots, diced
- 2 celery stalks, diced
- 4 cloves garlic, minced
- 1 tsp cumin
- 1 tsp smoked paprika
- 6 cups vegetable broth
- Salt and pepper to taste
- 2 tbsp lemon juice
- Chopped parsley for garnish

Instructions:
1. In a large pot, combine lentils, onion, carrots, celery, garlic, cumin, smoked paprika and vegetable broth.

2. Bring to a boil, then reduce heat and simmer for 30-40 minutes until lentils are tender.
3. Use an immersion blender to partially puree the soup for a thicker texture, if desired.
4. Season with salt, pepper and lemon juice.
5. Garnish with chopped parsley before serving.

Nutritional Information (per serving):
Calories: 180
Protein: 11g
Carbs: 30g
Fiber: 12g
Fat: 1g

Tofu Stir-Fry

Prep Time: 20 minutes
Cook Time: 15 minutes
Serves: 4

Ingredients:
- 14 oz extra-firm tofu, drained and cubed
- 2 tablespoons soy sauce or tamari
- 1 tablespoon rice vinegar

- 1 teaspoon sesame oil
- 2 tablespoons vegetable oil
- 1 red bell pepper, sliced
- 1 cup broccoli florets
- 1 cup sliced mushrooms
- 3 cloves garlic, minced
- 1 teaspoon grated ginger
- 2 green onions, sliced
- Cooked brown rice or quinoa, for serving

Instructions:
1. In a shallow dish, combine the tofu, soy sauce, rice vinegar, and sesame oil. Toss to coat and let marinate for 15 minutes.
2. Heat the vegetable oil in a large skillet or wok over high heat.
3. Add the marinated tofu and stir-fry for 5 minutes until lightly browned.
4. Add the bell pepper, broccoli, mushrooms, garlic, and ginger. Stir-fry for 5-7 minutes until vegetables are tender-crisp.
5. Add the green onions and toss to combine.
6. Serve hot over cooked brown rice or quinoa.

Nutritional Information (per serving):
Calories: 240

Protein: 14g
Carbs: 16g
Fiber: 4g
Fat: 13g

Eggplant and Chickpea Curry

Prep Time: 15 minutes
Cook Time: 30 minutes
Serves: 4

Ingredients:
- 1 large eggplant, cubed
- 1 (15 oz) can chickpeas, drained and rinsed
- 1 onion, diced
- 3 cloves garlic, minced
- 1 tablespoon grated ginger
- 1 tablespoon curry powder
- 1 teaspoon ground cumin
- 1 (14 oz) can diced tomatoes
- 1 cup vegetable broth
- 1/2 cup coconut milk
- Salt and pepper to taste
- Chopped cilantro for garnish

Instructions:
1. In a large skillet or Dutch oven, sauté the onion in 1 tablespoon of oil over medium heat until translucent, about 5 minutes.
2. Add the garlic, ginger, curry powder, and cumin. Cook for 1 minute until fragrant.
3. Add the eggplant, chickpeas, diced tomatoes, vegetable broth, and coconut milk. Season with salt and pepper.
4. Bring to a simmer and cook for 20-25 minutes, until the eggplant is tender.
5. Adjust seasoning if needed and garnish with chopped cilantro.
6. Serve over basmati rice or with naan bread.

Nutritional Information (per serving):
Calories: 290
Protein: 10g
Carbs: 44g
Fiber: 13g
Fat: 10g

Quinoa Stuffed Bell Peppers

Prep Time: 20 minutes
Cook Time: 40 minutes
Serves: 4

Ingredients:
- 4 bell peppers (any color), tops cut off and seeded
- 1 cup quinoa, rinsed
- 2 cups vegetable broth
- 1 (15oz) can black beans, drained and rinsed
- 1 cup corn kernels (fresh or frozen)
- 1/2 cup salsa
- 1 teaspoon cumin
- 1 teaspoon chili powder
- Salt and pepper to taste
- 1 cup shredded vegan cheese (optional)

Instructions:
1. Preheat oven to 375°F (190°C).
2. In a saucepan, bring the quinoa and vegetable broth to a boil. Reduce heat, cover and simmer for 15-20 minutes until quinoa is cooked.

3. In a bowl, mix cooked quinoa with black beans, corn, salsa, cumin, chili powder, salt and pepper.
4. Stuff the bell pepper cavities evenly with the quinoa mixture.
5. Place stuffed peppers in a baking dish and add 1/4 cup water or broth to the bottom.
6. Cover with foil and bake for 30 minutes. Remove foil, top with vegan cheese if using, and bake 10 more minutes.

Nutritional Info (per stuffed pepper):
Calories: 300
Protein: 12g
Carbs: 55g
Fiber: 11g
Fat: 3g

Vegetable and Lentil Shepherd's Pie

Prep Time: 20 minutes
Cook Time: 1 hour
Serves: 6

Ingredients:
- 1 cup dried green lentils
- 4 cups vegetable broth
- 2 carrots, diced
- 2 celery stalks, diced
- 1 onion, diced
- 2 cloves garlic, minced
- 1 tsp dried thyme
- 3 cups mashed potatoes
- 1 cup frozen peas
- Salt and pepper to taste

Instructions:
1. In a saucepan, combine lentils and broth. Bring to a boil, reduce heat and simmer for 20 minutes.
2. In a skillet, sauté the carrots, celery, onion and garlic for 5-7 minutes until soft.
3. Add cooked lentils with remaining broth and thyme. Season with salt and pepper.
4. Transfer to a baking dish and top with mashed potatoes, spreading evenly.
5. Top with frozen peas and bake at 375°F (190°C) for 30 minutes until heated through.

Nutritional Info (per serving):
Calories: 240

Protein: 12g
Carbs: 43g
Fiber: 10g
Fat: 1g

Spinach and Mushroom Quesadillas

Prep Time: 15 minutes
Cook Time: 10 minutes
Serves: 4

Ingredients:
- 8 small whole wheat tortillas
- 2 cups fresh spinach, chopped
- 1 cup sliced mushrooms
- 1/2 cup diced onion
- 1 clove garlic, minced
- 1 cup shredded vegan cheese
- 1 avocado, sliced
- Salsa for serving

Instructions:
1. In a skillet, sauté the mushrooms, onion and garlic for 3-4 minutes until soft.

2. Add the chopped spinach and cook for 1-2 more minutes until wilted. Season with salt and pepper.
3. Layer half the tortillas with the spinach/mushroom mixture and vegan cheese. Top with remaining tortillas.
4. Cook quesadillas for 2-3 minutes per side in a skillet or griddle over medium heat until crispy and cheese melts.
5. Slice into wedges and serve with avocado slices and salsa.

Nutritional Info (per quesadilla):
Calories: 320
Protein: 14g
Carbs: 43g
Fiber: 8g
Fat: 12g

Sweet Potato and Black Bean Tacos

Prep Time: 15 minutes
Cook Time: 30 minutes
Serves: 4

Ingredients:
- 2 medium sweet potatoes, peeled and diced
- 1 (15oz) can black beans, drained and rinsed
- 1 teaspoon cumin
- 1 teaspoon chili powder
- 1 teaspoon smoked paprika
- 8 small corn tortillas
- 1 avocado, sliced
- 1/4 cup diced red onion
- 2 tablespoons chopped cilantro
- Lime wedges for serving

Instructions:
1. Preheat oven to 400°F (200°C).
2. Toss the diced sweet potatoes with 1 tbsp olive oil, cumin, chili powder and smoked paprika on a baking sheet.
3. Roast for 20-25 minutes until potatoes are tender.
4. In a skillet, heat the black beans until warmed through.
5. Warm the tortillas according to package instructions.
6. Fill each tortilla with roasted sweet potatoes and warm black beans.
7. Top with avocado slices, diced red onion and cilantro.

8. Serve with lime wedges.

Nutritional Info (per 2 tacos):
Calories: 300
Protein: 10g
Carbs: 52g
Fiber: 13g
Fat: 8g

Zucchini Noodles with Pesto

Prep Time: 15 minutes
Cook Time: 5 minutes
Serves: 4

Ingredients:
- 4 medium zucchinis, spiralized into noodles
- 1 cup basil pesto (see recipe below)
- 1 pint cherry tomatoes, halved
- 1/4 cup toasted pine nuts

Basil Pesto:
- 2 cups fresh basil leaves
- 1/2 cup olive oil

- 1/3 cup pine nuts
- 3 garlic cloves
- 1/4 cup nutritional yeast
- Salt and pepper to taste

Instructions:
1. Make the pesto by blending all ingredients in a food processor until smooth.
2. In a large skillet, sauté the zucchini noodles for 2-3 minutes until just tender.
3. Remove from heat and toss with the pesto until noodles are well coated.
4. Stir in the cherry tomatoes and toasted pine nuts.
5. Serve immediately while zucchini noodles are still slightly crisp.

Nutritional Info (per serving):
Calories: 350
Protein: 9g
Carbs: 16g
Fiber: 4g
Fat: 30g

Pudding with Berries (Vegan)

Prep Time: 5 minutes
Chill Time: 2 hours
Serves: 4

Ingredients:
- 1 cup unsweetened almond milk
- 1/2 cup chia seeds
- 1/4 cup maple syrup
- 1 tsp vanilla extract
- 1 cup mixed berries

Instructions:
1. In a bowl, whisk together the almond milk, chia seeds, maple syrup and vanilla.
2. Let sit for 5 minutes, then whisk again to prevent clumping.
3. Cover and refrigerate for at least 2 hours to allow chia to thicken into a pudding.
4. Portion pudding into bowls or glasses and top with fresh berries before serving.

Nutritional Info (per serving):
Calories: 180

Protein: 5g
Carbs: 28g
Fiber: 10g
Fat: 7g

Vegan Lentil Sloppy Joes

Prep Time: 10 minutes
Cook Time: 30 minutes
Serves: 4

Ingredients:
- 1 cup dried brown or green lentils, rinsed
- 3 cups vegetable broth or water
- 1 tbsp olive oil
- 1 onion, diced
- 2 cloves garlic, minced
- 1 cup diced bell pepper
- 1 cup diced mushrooms
- 1 (15oz) can tomato sauce
- 2 tbsp tomato paste
- 2 tbsp vegan Worcestershire sauce
- 1 tbsp brown sugar (optional)

- 1 tsp chili powder
- Salt and pepper to taste
- 4 whole wheat burger buns

Instructions:
1. In a saucepan, combine the lentils and broth/water. Bring to a boil, reduce heat and simmer for 20 minutes until lentils are tender. Drain excess liquid.
2. In a skillet, heat the olive oil over medium heat. Sauté the onion for 2-3 minutes until translucent.
3. Add the garlic, bell pepper and mushrooms. Cook for 5 more minutes.
4. Stir in the cooked lentils, tomato sauce, tomato paste, Worcestershire, brown sugar, chili powder and season with salt and pepper.
5. Simmer for 10 minutes to allow flavors to blend.
6. Serve warm lentil mixture on toasted buns.

Nutritional Info (per serving):
Calories: 310
Protein: 15g
Carbs: 53g
Fiber: 16g
Fat: 4g

Cauliflower and Chickpea Curry

Prep Time: 15 minutes
Cook Time: 30 minutes
Serves: 4

Ingredients:
- 1 head cauliflower, cut into florets
- 1 (15oz) can chickpeas, drained and rinsed
- 1 onion, diced
- 3 cloves garlic, minced
- 1 tbsp grated ginger
- 2 tsp garam masala
- 1 tsp cumin
- 1 tsp turmeric
- 1 (14oz) can diced tomatoes
- 1 cup vegetable broth
- 1/2 cup coconut milk
- Salt and pepper to taste
- Chopped cilantro for garnish

Instructions:
1. In a large pot or dutch oven, sauté the onions in 1 tbsp oil over medium heat for 2-3 minutes.

2. Add the garlic, ginger, garam masala, cumin and turmeric. Cook for 1 minute until fragrant.
3. Stir in the cauliflower, chickpeas, diced tomatoes and vegetable broth. Season with salt and pepper.
4. Bring to a simmer and cook for 15-20 minutes until cauliflower is tender.
5. Stir in the coconut milk and adjust seasoning as needed.
6. Garnish with chopped cilantro and serve over basmati rice.

Nutritional Info (per serving):
Calories: 280
Protein: 12g
Carbs: 38g
Fiber: 12g
Fat: 11g

Mushroom and Spinach Quinoa Pilaf

Prep Time: 10 minutes
Cook Time: 25 minutes
Serves: 4

Ingredients:
- 1 cup quinoa, rinsed
- 2 cups vegetable broth
- 8oz sliced mushrooms
- 2 cloves garlic, minced
- 2 cups fresh spinach
- 1/4 cup sliced almonds
- 2 tbsp lemon juice
- Salt and pepper to taste

Instructions:
1. In a saucepan, combine the quinoa and vegetable broth. Bring to a boil, then reduce heat and simmer covered for 15 minutes.
2. In a skillet, sauté the mushrooms in 1 tbsp olive oil for 5 minutes until browned. Add garlic and cook 1 minute more.
3. Stir in the cooked quinoa, spinach, almonds, lemon juice and season with salt and pepper to taste.
4. Cook for 2-3 minutes until spinach is wilted.

Nutritional Info (per serving):
Calories: 220
Protein: 8g
Carbs: 33g
Fiber: 5g

Fat: 7g

Vegan Chili

Prep Time: 15 minutes
Cook Time: 45 minutes
Serves: 6

Ingredients:
- 1 tbsp olive oil
- 1 onion, diced
- 3 cloves garlic, minced
- 1 jalapeño, seeded and minced (optional)
- 2 tbsp chili powder
- 2 tsp ground cumin
- 1 tsp smoked paprika
- 1 (28oz) can crushed tomatoes
- 1 (15oz) can kidney beans, drained and rinsed
- 1 (15oz) can black beans, drained and rinsed
- 1 cup vegetable broth
- Salt and pepper to taste
- Chopped cilantro, avocado, lime wedges for serving

Instructions:
1. In a large pot, heat the olive oil over medium heat. Sauté the onion for 3-4 minutes until translucent.
2. Add the garlic, jalapeño, chili powder, cumin and paprika. Cook for 1 minute until fragrant.
3. Stir in the crushed tomatoes, kidney beans, black beans, and vegetable broth. Season with salt and pepper.
4. Bring to a boil, then reduce heat and simmer for 30 minutes, stirring occasionally.
5. Adjust seasoning to taste. Serve hot topped with cilantro, avocado and lime wedges.

Nutritional Info (per serving):
Calories: 240
Protein: 12g
Carbs: 42g
Fiber: 13g
Fat: 4g

Stuffed Portobello Mushrooms

Prep Time: 15 minutes

Cook Time: 25 minutes
Serves: 4

Ingredients:
- 4 large portobello mushroom caps
- 1 cup cooked quinoa
- 1/2 cup diced bell pepper
- 1/2 cup diced onion
- 2 cloves garlic, minced
- 1 cup fresh spinach, chopped
- 1/2 cup breadcrumbs
- 1/4 cup grated vegan parmesan
- 2 tbsp olive oil
- Salt and pepper to taste

Instructions:
1. Preheat oven to 375°F (190°C). Remove stems from mushroom caps and scoop out some interior to create a cavity.
2. In a skillet, sauté the onion and bell pepper in 1 tbsp olive oil for 3-4 minutes.
3. Add the garlic and spinach and cook 1 minute until wilted.
4. In a bowl, mix the cooked quinoa, sautéed veggies, breadcrumbs, vegan parmesan and

remaining 1 tbsp olive oil. Season with salt and pepper.

5. Stuff the mushroom caps evenly with the quinoa mixture.

6. Arrange stuffed mushrooms cap-side up in a baking dish and bake for 20-25 minutes until mushrooms are tender.

Nutritional Info (per stuffed mushroom):
Calories: 180
Protein: 6g
Carbs: 24g
Fiber: 4g
Fat: 8g

Tofu Scramble Breakfast Tacos

Prep Time: 10 minutes
Cook Time: 10 minutes
Serves: 4

Ingredients:
- 1 (14oz) package firm tofu, drained and crumbled

- 1 tbsp olive oil
- 1/2 onion, diced
- 1 bell pepper, diced
- 1 cup sliced mushrooms
- 2 tsp turmeric
- 1 tsp cumin
- 1 tsp garlic powder
- Salt and pepper to taste
- 8 small corn tortillas
- Toppings: avocado, salsa, vegan cheese shreds

Instructions:
1. In a skillet, heat the olive oil over medium heat. Sauté the onion for 2-3 minutes until translucent.
2. Add the bell pepper and mushrooms and cook for 5 minutes more.
3. Crumble in the tofu and sprinkle with turmeric, cumin, garlic powder, salt and pepper. Cook for 3-4 minutes, stirring often.
4. Warm the tortillas according to package instructions.
5. Fill each tortilla with a scoop of the tofu scramble. Top with avocado, salsa, vegan cheese if desired.

Nutritional Info (per 2 tacos):

Calories: 290
Protein: 15g
Carbs: 32g
Fiber: 7g
Fat: 12g

Vegan Pad Thai

Prep Time: 20 minutes
Cook Time: 15 minutes
Serves: 4

Ingredients:
- 8 oz rice noodles
- 2 tbsp sesame oil
- 3 cloves garlic, minced
- 1-inch ginger, grated
- 1 cup shredded carrots
- 1 cup bean sprouts
- 1/2 cup sliced green onions
- 1/4 cup soy sauce
- 2 tbsp rice vinegar
- 2 tbsp brown sugar

- 1 tbsp sriracha (or to taste)
- 1/4 cup chopped cilantro
- 1/4 cup chopped peanuts

Instructions:
1. Cook rice noodles according to package instructions. Drain and rinse with cold water to stop cooking. Set aside.
2. In a large skillet or wok, heat sesame oil over medium-high heat. Add garlic and ginger, cook for 1 minute.
3. Add carrots and bean sprouts, stir-fry for 2 minutes.
4. Add cooked noodles, soy sauce, vinegar, brown sugar and sriracha. Toss everything together for 2-3 minutes.
5. Remove from heat and stir in green onions and cilantro.
6. Serve immediately, garnished with chopped peanuts.

Nutritional Info (per serving):
Calories: 370
Protein: 8g
Carbs: 63g
Fiber: 4g

Fat: 11g

Veggie and Hummus Wrap

Prep Time: 10 minutes
Serves: 2

Ingredients:
- 2 large whole wheat tortillas or wraps
- 1/2 cup hummus
- 1 cup shredded lettuce
- 1/2 cucumber, sliced
- 1/2 bell pepper, sliced
- 1/4 cup shredded carrots
- 1/4 cup sliced red onion
- 2 tbsp olive tapenade (optional)

Instructions:
1. Lay the tortillas on a flat surface and spread 1/4 cup hummus down the center of each.
2. Top with shredded lettuce, cucumber, bell pepper, carrots and red onion.
3. Drizzle with olive tapenade if using.

4. Fold the bottom of the tortilla over the filling, then fold in the sides and continue rolling up tightly.
5. Slice in half to serve.

Nutritional Info (per wrap):
Calories: 330
Protein: 12g
Carbs: 46g
Fiber: 10g
Fat: 14g

Poultry, Meat and Potatoes

Here are some poultry, meat and potato options with preparation time, cooking time, ingredients, instructions and nutritional information:

Lemon Herb Baked Chicken

Prep Time: 10 minutes
Cook Time: 40 minutes
Servings: 4

Ingredients:

- 4 boneless, skinless chicken breasts
- 2 tbsp olive oil
- 1 tsp dried basil
- 1 tsp dried oregano
- 1/2 tsp garlic powder
- Zest of 1 lemon
- Salt and pepper to taste
- 1 lemon, sliced

Instructions:
1. Preheat oven to 400°F (200°C).
2. In a small bowl, combine olive oil, dried herbs, garlic powder, lemon zest, salt, and pepper.
3. Pat chicken breasts dry and place in a baking dish. Rub the herb mixture all over the chicken.
4. Arrange lemon slices around the chicken.
5. Bake for 35-40 minutes, or until chicken is cooked through (internal temperature of 165°F/74°C).
6. Let rest for 5 minutes before serving.

Nutritional Value (per serving):
Calories: 220, Protein: 38g, Carbs: 2g, Fiber: 0g, Fat: 8g

Beef and Broccoli Stir-Fry

Prep Time: 15 minutes
Cook Time: 15 minutes
Servings: 4

Ingredients:
- 1 lb sirloin steak, thinly sliced
- 2 tbsp olive oil, divided
- 4 cups broccoli florets
- 1 red bell pepper, sliced
- 1 onion, sliced
- 3 cloves garlic, minced
- 2 tbsp soy sauce
- 1 tsp sesame oil
- Salt and pepper to taste
- Cooked rice or noodles, for serving

Instructions:
1. In a large skillet or wok, heat 1 tbsp olive oil over high heat. Add sliced beef and stir-fry until browned but not fully cooked, about 2-3 minutes. Transfer to a plate.

2. Add remaining 1 tbsp olive oil to the skillet. Add broccoli, bell pepper, onion, and garlic. Stir-fry for 5-7 minutes until vegetables are tender-crisp.
3. Return beef and its juices to the skillet. Add soy sauce and sesame oil. Toss to combine.
4. Season with salt and pepper to taste.
5. Serve immediately over rice or noodles.

Nutritional Value (per serving):
Calories: 330, Protein: 28g, Carbs: 12g, Fiber: 3g, Fat: 19g

Roasted Sweet Potato Wedges

Prep Time: 10 minutes
Cook Time: 30 minutes
Servings: 4

Ingredients:
- 2 large sweet potatoes, cut into wedges
- 2 tbsp olive oil
- 1 tsp paprika
- 1 tsp garlic powder
- 1/2 tsp salt

- 1/4 tsp black pepper
- Chopped fresh parsley for garnish

Instructions:
1. Preheat oven to 425°F (220°C). Line a baking sheet with parchment paper or foil.
2. In a large bowl, toss the sweet potato wedges with olive oil, paprika, garlic powder, salt, and pepper until evenly coated.
3. Spread the wedges in a single layer on the prepared baking sheet.
4. Roast for 25-30 minutes, flipping halfway, until tender and lightly browned.
5. Garnish with fresh parsley before serving.

Nutritional Value (per serving):
Calories: 160, Protein: 2g, Carbs: 21g, Fiber: 4g, Fat: 8g

Shepherd's Pie

Prep Time: 20 minutes
Cook Time: 45 minutes
Servings: 6

Ingredients:
- 1 lb ground beef or lamb
- 1 onion, diced
- 2 carrots, diced
- 2 cups frozen peas
- 2 tbsp tomato paste
- 1 cup beef broth
- 1 tsp Worcestershire sauce
- Salt and pepper to taste
- 3 cups mashed potatoes
- 1/2 cup shredded cheddar cheese

Instructions:
1. Preheat oven to 375°F (190°C).
2. In a skillet over medium heat, cook the ground beef or lamb until browned and crumbled. Drain excess fat.
3. Add onions and carrots to the skillet. Cook for 5 minutes until softened.
4. Stir in peas, tomato paste, beef broth, Worcestershire sauce, salt, and pepper. Simmer for 10 minutes.
5. Transfer the meat mixture to a baking dish.
6. Spread the mashed potatoes evenly over the top.
7. Sprinkle with shredded cheddar cheese.

8. Bake for 25-30 minutes, or until the potatoes are golden brown.
9. Let cool for 5 minutes before serving.

Nutritional Value (per serving):
Calories: 410, Protein: 22g, Carbs: 39g, Fiber: 5g, Fat: 18g

Turkey Meatballs with Zucchini Noodles

Prep Time: 20 minutes
Cook Time: 20 minutes
Servings: 4

Ingredients:
- 1 lb ground turkey
- 1 egg
- 1/2 cup breadcrumbs
- 1/4 cup grated Parmesan cheese
- 2 cloves garlic, minced
- 1 tsp Italian seasoning
- Salt and pepper to taste
- 2 zucchinis, spiralized or julienned
- 2 cups marinara sauce

Instructions:
1. Preheat oven to 400°F (200°C). Line a baking sheet with parchment paper.
2. In a bowl, mix together ground turkey, egg, breadcrumbs, Parmesan, garlic, Italian seasoning, salt, and pepper until well combined.
3. Roll the mixture into 1-inch meatballs and place them on the prepared baking sheet.
4. Bake for 15-18 minutes, or until cooked through.
5. While meatballs are baking, spiralize or julienne the zucchinis.
6. Heat marinara sauce in a skillet over medium heat.
7. Add the zucchini noodles and cooked meatballs to the marinara sauce. Toss to combine and cook for 2-3 minutes until heated through.
8. Serve immediately.

Nutritional Value (per serving):
Calories: 370, Protein: 32g, Carbs: 27g, Fiber: 4g, Fat: 16g

Herb-Roasted Turkey Breast

Prep Time: 10 minutes
Cook Time: 1.5-2 hours
Serves: 6

Ingredients:
- 3 lb turkey breast, bone-in
- 3 tbsp olive oil
- 2 tsp dried thyme
- 2 tsp dried rosemary
- 1 tsp garlic powder
- 1 tsp salt
- 1/2 tsp black pepper

Instructions:
1. Preheat oven to 325°F.
2. Pat the turkey breast dry and rub all over with olive oil.
3. In a small bowl, mix together the thyme, rosemary, garlic powder, salt and pepper.
4. Rub the spice mixture all over the turkey breast.
5. Place breast side up on a rack in a roasting pan.

6. Roast for 1.5-2 hours until internal temperature reaches 165°F in the thickest part.
7. Let rest 15 minutes before slicing.

Nutritional Info (per 4oz serving):
Calories: 190
Protein: 25g
Carbs: 0g
Fat: 8g

Honey Mustard Glazed Chicken

Prep Time: 10 minutes
Cook Time: 30 minutes
Serves: 4

Ingredients:
- 4 boneless, skinless chicken breasts
- 1/4 cup Dijon mustard
- 2 tbsp honey
- 1 tbsp olive oil
- 1 tsp dried thyme
- 1/2 tsp salt
- 1/4 tsp black pepper

Instructions:

1. Preheat oven to 400°F. Lightly grease a baking dish.
2. In a small bowl, mix the mustard, honey, olive oil, thyme, salt and pepper.
3. Place chicken breasts in the prepared baking dish and coat with the honey mustard mixture.
4. Bake for 25-30 minutes until chicken is cooked through and juices run clear.
5. Spoon any extra sauce from the pan over the chicken before serving.

Nutrition (per breast):
Calories: 290
Protein: 38g
Carbs: 14g
Fat: 8g

Mediterranean Chicken Skewers

Prep Time: 20 minutes (plus 30 mins marinating)
Cook Time: 15 minutes
Serves: 4

Ingredients:
- 1 lb boneless, skinless chicken breasts, cut into 1-inch cubes
- 1/4 cup olive oil
- 2 tbsp lemon juice
- 2 cloves garlic, minced
- 1 tsp dried oregano
- 1 tsp dried basil
- 1/2 tsp salt
- 1/4 tsp black pepper
- 1 red bell pepper, cut into 1-inch pieces
- 1 red onion, cut into wedges

Instructions:
1. In a shallow dish, mix olive oil, lemon juice, garlic, oregano, basil, salt and pepper.
2. Add chicken and toss to coat. Cover and marinate for 30 minutes.
3. Thread chicken, bell pepper and onion alternately onto skewers.
4. Preheat grill or grill pan to medium-high heat. Grill skewers for 12-15 minutes, turning occasionally, until chicken is cooked through.

Nutrition (per 2 skewers):

Calories: 280
Protein: 28g
Carbs: 8g
Fat: 15g

Herb-Roasted Potatoes

Prep Time: 10 minutes
Cook Time: 40 minutes
Serves: 4

Ingredients:
- 1.5 lbs baby potatoes, halved
- 2 tbsp olive oil
- 1 tsp dried thyme
- 1 tsp dried rosemary
- 1/2 tsp garlic powder
- 1/2 tsp salt
- 1/4 tsp black pepper

Instructions:
1. Preheat oven to 400°F.

2. In a large bowl, toss the potatoes with olive oil, thyme, rosemary, garlic powder, salt and pepper until coated.

3. Arrange potatoes in a single layer on a baking sheet.

4. Roast for 35-40 minutes, stirring halfway, until potatoes are fork-tender and browned.

Nutrition (per serving):
Calories: 170
Protein: 3g
Carbs: 22g
Fat: 8g

Balsamic Glazed Salmon

Prep Time: 10 minutes
Marinate Time: 30 minutes
Cook Time: 12-15 minutes
Serves: 4

Ingredients:
- 4 (6oz) salmon fillets
- 1/4 cup balsamic vinegar

- 2 tbsp honey
- 2 tbsp olive oil
- 2 cloves garlic, minced
- 1 tsp dried basil
- 1/2 tsp salt
- 1/4 tsp black pepper

Instructions:
1. In a shallow dish, whisk together the balsamic vinegar, honey, olive oil, garlic, basil, salt and pepper.
2. Add the salmon fillets and turn to coat both sides with the marinade. Cover and marinate for 30 minutes in the fridge.
3. Preheat oven to 400°F. Line a baking sheet with foil.
4. Transfer salmon to the baking sheet and bake for 12-15 minutes, until salmon is opaque and flakes easily with a fork.

Nutrition (per 6oz fillet):
Calories: 370
Protein: 34g
Carbs: 16g
Fat: 19g

Garlic and Herb Steak

Prep Time: 5 minutes (plus 30 mins resting)
Cook Time: 10-15 minutes
Serves: 4

Ingredients:
- 1.5 lbs flank or skirt steak
- 3 tbsp olive oil
- 3 cloves garlic, minced
- 2 tsp dried rosemary
- 2 tsp dried thyme
- 1 tsp salt
- 1/2 tsp black pepper

Instructions:
1. Pat the steak dry and let it rest at room temperature for 30 minutes before cooking.
2. In a small bowl, mix together the olive oil, garlic, rosemary, thyme, salt and pepper.
3. Rub the garlic-herb mixture all over the steak on both sides.

4. Preheat grill or grill pan to high heat. Grill steak for 5-7 minutes per side for medium-rare, or until desired doneness.

5. Transfer steak to a cutting board and let rest 5 minutes before slicing against the grain.

Nutrition (per 6oz serving):
Calories: 450
Protein: 40g
Carbs: 1g
Fat: 32g

Sweet Potato and Black Bean Hash

Prep Time: 10 minutes
Cook Time: 25 minutes
Serves: 4

Ingredients:
- 2 tbsp olive oil
- 1 onion, diced
- 1 bell pepper, diced
- 2 large sweet potatoes, peeled and cubed
- 1 (15oz) can black beans, drained and rinsed

- 2 tsp cumin
- 1 tsp smoked paprika
- 1/2 tsp salt
- 1/4 tsp black pepper
- 2 tbsp chopped cilantro

Instructions:
1. Heat the olive oil in a large skillet over medium-high heat.
2. Add the onion and bell pepper and cook for 3 minutes until starting to soften.
3. Add the sweet potato cubes and cook for 10 minutes, stirring occasionally, until potatoes are tender.
4. Stir in the black beans, cumin, smoked paprika, salt and pepper.
5. Continue cooking for 5 more minutes to heat through and allow flavors to blend.
6. Remove from heat and stir in chopped cilantro.

Nutrition (per serving):
Calories: 290
Protein: 8g
Carbs: 44g
Fiber: 10g
Fat: 9g

Mashed Cauliflower and Garlic Potatoes

Prep Time: 15 minutes
Cook Time: 20 minutes
Serves: 4

Ingredients:
- 1 head cauliflower, cut into florets
- 1 lb Yukon Gold potatoes, peeled and cubed
- 1/2 cup milk (dairy or plant-based)
- 2 tbsp butter or olive oil
- 4 cloves garlic, minced
- 1/2 tsp salt
- 1/4 tsp black pepper
- 2 tbsp chopped chives for garnish

Instructions:
1. In a large pot, bring salted water to a boil. Add cauliflower and potato cubes. Cook for 15-20 minutes until very tender.
2. Drain well and return to the pot.

3. Add milk, butter/olive oil and garlic. Mash with a potato masher or hand mixer until smooth and creamy.
4. Season with salt and pepper.
5. Garnish with chopped chives before serving.

Nutrition (per serving):
Calories: 200
Protein: 6g
Carbs: 29g
Fiber: 6g
Fat: 8g

Roasted Fingerling Potatoes

Prep Time: 10 minutes
Cook Time: 30 minutes
Serves: 4

Ingredients:
- 1.5 lbs fingerling potatoes, halved lengthwise
- 2 tbsp olive oil
- 2 tsp fresh rosemary, chopped
- 2 cloves garlic, minced

- 1 tsp salt
- 1/2 tsp black pepper

Instructions:
1. Preheat oven to 425°F. Line a baking sheet with parchment paper.
2. In a large bowl, toss the potatoes with olive oil, rosemary, garlic, salt and pepper until coated.
3. Arrange potatoes in a single layer on the prepared baking sheet.
4. Roast for 25-30 minutes, stirring halfway, until potatoes are fork-tender and browned.

Nutrition (per serving):
Calories: 220
Protein: 3g
Carbs: 28g
Fiber: 3g
Fat: 10g

Greek Potato Salad

Prep Time: 15 minutes
Cook Time: 15 minutes

Serves: 4

Ingredients:
- 1.5 lbs baby potatoes, halved
- 1/4 cup olive oil
- 2 tbsp red wine vinegar
- 1 tsp Dijon mustard
- 1/2 red onion, thinly sliced
- 1 cup cherry tomatoes, halved
- 1/2 cup Kalamata olives, pitted and halved
- 1/4 cup crumbled feta cheese
- 2 tbsp chopped fresh parsley

Instructions:
1. In a pot of salted water, boil the potatoes for 12-15 minutes until fork-tender. Drain and let cool slightly.
2. Make the dressing by whisking the olive oil, red wine vinegar and Dijon mustard.
3. In a large bowl, toss the cooked potatoes with the dressing.
4. Add the red onion, tomatoes, olives, feta and parsley. Toss gently to combine.
5. Refrigerate for 30 minutes before serving to allow flavors to blend.

Nutrition (per serving):
Calories: 340
Protein: 5g
Carbs: 31g
Fiber: 4g
Fat: 22g

Ginger Soy Glazed Pork Chops

Prep Time: 10 minutes (plus 30 mins marinating)
Cook Time: 15 minutes
Serves: 4

Ingredients:
- 4 (6oz) boneless pork chops
- 1/4 cup low-sodium soy sauce
- 2 tbsp rice vinegar
- 2 tbsp honey
- 1 tbsp sesame oil
- 1 tbsp freshly grated ginger
- 2 cloves garlic, minced
- 1 tbsp olive oil

Instructions:

1. In a shallow dish, whisk together the soy sauce, rice vinegar, honey, sesame oil, ginger and garlic. Add the pork chops and turn to coat both sides. Cover and marinate for 30 minutes.
2. Heat the olive oil in a large skillet over medium-high heat.
3. Remove pork chops from marinade (reserve marinade) and cook for 4-5 minutes per side until browned and cooked through.
4. Transfer pork chops to a plate and tent with foil.
5. Add reserved marinade to the skillet and simmer for 2-3 minutes until thickened into a glaze.
6. Pour glaze over pork chops and serve.

Nutritional Information (per chop):
Calories: 320
Protein: 26g
Carbs: 16g
Fat: 16g

Turmeric Lamb Kabobs

Prep Time: 20 minutes (plus 30 mins marinating)

Cook Time: 12 minutes
Serves: 4

Ingredients:
- 1 lb boneless lamb shoulder, cut into 1-inch cubes
- 1/4 cup olive oil
- 2 tbsp lemon juice
- 4 cloves garlic, minced
- 1 tbsp ground turmeric
- 1 tsp ground cumin
- 1 tsp paprika
- 1 tsp salt
- 1/2 tsp black pepper
- Metal or wooden skewers

Instructions:
1. In a shallow dish, whisk together olive oil, lemon juice, garlic, turmeric, cumin, paprika, salt and pepper.
2. Add the lamb cubes and toss to coat. Cover and marinate for 30 minutes.
3. Thread lamb cubes onto skewers, leaving a little space between each cube.
4. Preheat grill or grill pan to medium-high heat. Grill kabobs for 10-12 minutes, turning occasionally, until lamb is cooked through.

Nutritional Information (per 2 kabobs):
Calories: 370
Protein: 24g
Carbs: 2g
Fat: 29g

Chili Lime Shrimp Tacos

Prep Time: 15 minutes
Cook Time: 5 minutes
Serves: 4

Ingredients:
- 1 lb large shrimp, peeled and deveined
- 2 tbsp olive oil
- 1 tbsp lime juice
- 1 tsp chili powder
- 1/2 tsp cumin
- 1/4 tsp cayenne pepper
- Salt and pepper to taste
- 8 small corn tortillas, warmed
- Shredded cabbage, diced avocado, lime wedges for serving

Instructions:

1. In a bowl, toss the shrimp with olive oil, lime juice, chili powder, cumin, cayenne and season with salt and pepper.
2. Heat a skillet over high heat. Add the shrimp in a single layer and cook for 2-3 minutes per side until opaque and cooked through.
3. Warm the tortillas according to package instructions.
4. Fill each tortilla with shrimp, shredded cabbage, avocado and a squeeze of lime juice.

Nutritional Information (per 2 tacos):
Calories: 250
Protein: 20g
Carbs: 24g
Fat: 10g

Sauces, Condiments and Dressings

Here are the sauces, condiments, and dressings with preparation time, cooking time, ingredients, instructions, and nutritional information:

Almond Butter

Prep Time: 5 minutes
Cook Time: None

Ingredients:
- 2 cups raw almonds
- 1/4 tsp salt (optional)
- 1-2 tbsp coconut oil or avocado oil (optional)

Instructions:
1. Preheat oven to 350°F (175°C).
2. Spread the almonds on a baking sheet and roast for 8-10 minutes, stirring occasionally, until fragrant and lightly golden.
3. Let the roasted almonds cool completely.
4. Transfer the almonds to a high-powered blender or food processor. Blend/process for 5-10 minutes, stopping to scrape down the sides as needed, until a smooth and creamy butter forms.
5. If the mixture seems dry or isn't blending well, add 1-2 tbsp of coconut oil or avocado oil.

6. Add salt to taste, if desired.
7. Transfer the almond butter to an airtight container and store at room temperature for up to 2 weeks.

Nutritional Value (per 2 tbsp serving):
Calories: 195, Protein: 6g, Carbs: 6g, Fiber: 3g, Fat: 18g

Balsamic Vinaigrette

Prep Time: 5 minutes
Cook Time: None

Ingredients:
- 1/2 cup olive oil
- 1/4 cup balsamic vinegar
- 1 tbsp Dijon mustard
- 1 clove garlic, minced
- 1 tsp honey or maple syrup
- Salt and pepper to taste

Instructions:
1. In a small bowl or jar, whisk together (or shake) all the ingredients until well combined and emulsified.

2. Taste and adjust seasoning with salt and pepper as needed.
3. Store any leftovers in the refrigerator for up to 1 week.

Nutritional Value (per 2 tbsp serving):
Calories: 170, Protein: 0g, Carbs: 3g, Fiber: 0g, Fat: 18g

Guacamole

Prep Time: 10 minutes
Cook Time: None

Ingredients:
- 3 ripe avocados, pitted and mashed
- 1/4 cup diced red onion
- 1 jalapeño, seeded and minced (optional)
- 2 tbsp chopped fresh cilantro
- 2 tbsp lime juice
- 1/2 tsp salt
- 1/4 tsp ground cumin

Instructions:

1. In a medium bowl, mash the avocados with a fork or potato masher until slightly chunky.
2. Add the diced onion, jalapeño (if using), cilantro, lime juice, salt, and cumin. Mix well to combine.
3. Taste and adjust seasoning as needed.
4. Cover with plastic wrap, pressing it directly onto the surface of the guacamole to prevent browning.
5. Refrigerate for up to 2 days.

Nutritional Value (per 1/4 cup serving):
Calories: 120, Protein: 1g, Carbs: 6g, Fiber: 4g, Fat: 11g

Taco Seasoning

Prep Time: 5 minutes
Cook Time: None

Ingredients:
- 1 tbsp chili powder
- 1 tsp ground cumin
- 1 tsp paprika
- 1/2 tsp garlic powder
- 1/2 tsp onion powder
- 1/2 tsp dried oregano

- 1/4 tsp cayenne pepper (optional)
- 1 tsp salt
- 1/2 tsp black pepper

Instructions:
1. In a small bowl, mix together all the spices until well combined.
2. Store the taco seasoning in an airtight container at room temperature for up to 6 months.
3. To use, add 2-3 tbsp of the seasoning mix to 1 lb of ground beef, turkey, or plant-based protein crumbles when cooking.

Nutritional Value (per 1 tbsp serving):
Calories: 20, Protein: 1g, Carbs: 3g, Fiber: 2g, Fat: 1g

Lemon Tahini Dressing

Prep Time: 5 minutes
Cook Time: None

Ingredients:
- 1/4 cup tahini
- 1/4 cup lemon juice

- 2 tbsp olive oil
- 2 tbsp water (or more for desired consistency)
- 1 clove garlic, minced
- 1 tsp honey or maple syrup
- 1/4 tsp salt
- 1/4 tsp ground black pepper

Instructions:
1. In a small bowl or jar, whisk together (or shake) all the ingredients until well combined and emulsified.
2. If the dressing seems too thick, add more water 1 tbsp at a time until desired consistency is reached.
3. Taste and adjust seasoning as needed.
4. Store any leftovers in the refrigerator for up to 5 days.

Nutritional Value (per 2 tbsp serving):
Calories: 130, Protein: 2g, Carbs: 4g, Fiber: 1g, Fat: 12g

Avocado Cilantro Lime Sauce

Prep Time: 10 minutes
Cook Time: 0 minutes

Ingredients:
- 1 ripe avocado
- 1/4 cup cilantro leaves
- 2 tablespoons lime juice
- 1 garlic clove
- 1/4 cup water
- 1/2 teaspoon salt

Instructions:
1. In a blender or food processor, blend all ingredients until smooth and creamy.
2. Add more water if needed to reach desired consistency.

Nutritional Information (per 1/4 cup serving):
Calories: 92, Fat: 8g, Carbs: 5g, Protein: 1g

Garlic-Herb Yogurt Sauce

Prep Time: 10 minutes
Cook Time: 0 minutes

Ingredients:
- 1 cup plain Greek yogurt
- 2 tablespoons olive oil

- 2 garlic cloves, minced
- 2 tablespoons fresh parsley, chopped
- 1 tablespoon fresh dill, chopped
- 1 tablespoon lemon juice
- 1/2 teaspoon salt
- 1/4 teaspoon black pepper

Instructions:
1. In a small bowl, mix together the yogurt, olive oil, garlic, parsley, dill, lemon juice, salt and pepper until well combined.
2. Let sit for 10 minutes to allow flavors to meld.

Nutritional Information (per 1/4 cup serving):
Calories: 73, Fat: 5g, Carbs: 2g, Protein: 5g

Roasted Red Pepper Pesto

Prep Time: 10 minutes
Cook Time: 0 minutes

Ingredients:
- 1 jar (12 oz) roasted red peppers, drained
- 1/2 cup toasted walnuts
- 1 garlic clove

- 1/4 cup olive oil
- 1/4 cup grated Parmesan cheese
- 2 tablespoons lemon juice
- 1/4 teaspoon salt

Instructions:
1. In a food processor, combine the red peppers, walnuts, garlic and olive oil. Process until finely chopped.
2. Add the Parmesan, lemon juice and salt. Pulse until just combined.

Nutritional Information (per 2 tbsp serving):
Calories: 99, Fat: 9g, Carbs: 3g, Protein: 2g

Lemon-Tahini Sauce

Prep Time: 5 minutes
Cook Time: 0 minutes

Ingredients:
- 1/2 cup tahini
- 1/4 cup lemon juice
- 1 garlic clove, minced
- 1/4 cup water

- 1 teaspoon maple syrup
- 1/2 teaspoon salt

Instructions:
1. In a small bowl, whisk together all ingredients until well combined.
2. If too thick, add more water 1-2 tablespoons at a time.

Nutritional Information (per 2 tbsp serving):
Calories: 85, Fat: 7g, Carbs: 4g, Protein: 2g

Cucumber Yogurt Sauce

Prep Time: 10 minutes
Cook Time: 0 minutes

Ingredients:
- 1 cup plain Greek yogurt
- 1/2 cucumber, grated
- 2 tablespoons fresh dill, chopped
- 1 garlic clove, minced
- 2 teaspoons lemon juice
- 1/2 teaspoon salt
- 1/4 teaspoon black pepper

Instructions:
1. In a small bowl, mix together the yogurt, grated cucumber, dill, garlic, lemon juice, salt and pepper until well combined.
2. Let sit for 10 minutes to allow flavors to meld.
3. Drain off any excess liquid before serving.

Nutritional Information (per 1/4 cup serving):
Calories: 35, Fat: 0g, Carbs: 3g, Protein: 5g

Balsamic Honey Glaze

Prep Time: 5 minutes
Cook Time: 5 minutes

Ingredients:
- 1/2 cup balsamic vinegar
- 2 tablespoons honey
- 1 tablespoon Dijon mustard
- 1 garlic clove, minced
- 1/4 teaspoon salt
- 1/4 teaspoon black pepper

Instructions:

1. In a small saucepan, whisk together all ingredients.
2. Bring to a simmer over medium heat and cook for 3-5 minutes, stirring frequently, until thickened.
3. Remove from heat and let cool slightly before using.

Nutritional Information (per 2 tbsp serving):
Calories: 43, Fat: 0g, Carbs: 11g, Protein: 0g

Green Dressing

Prep Time: 10 minutes
Cook Time: 0 minutes

Ingredients:
- 1 cup fresh parsley leaves
- 1/2 cup olive oil
- 1/4 cup red wine vinegar
- 2 tablespoons Dijon mustard
- 2 garlic cloves
- 1 teaspoon honey
- 1/2 teaspoon salt
- 1/4 teaspoon black pepper

Instructions:
1. In a blender, combine all ingredients and blend until smooth and creamy.
2. Adjust seasoning if needed.

Nutritional Information (per 2 tbsp serving):
Calories: 137, Fat: 14g, Carbs: 2g, Protein: 0g

Spicy Mango Salsa

Prep Time: 15 minutes
Cook Time: 0 minutes

Ingredients:
- 2 ripe mangoes, diced
- 1/2 red onion, diced
- 1 jalapeño, seeded and minced
- 1/4 cup fresh cilantro, chopped
- 2 tablespoons lime juice
- 1 garlic clove, minced
- 1/2 teaspoon salt

Instructions:

1. In a medium bowl, combine the diced mangoes, red onion, jalapeño, cilantro, lime juice, garlic, and salt.
2. Gently toss to combine all ingredients.
3. Let sit for 10-15 minutes to allow flavors to meld.
4. Serve with chips, tacos, or as a topping.

Nutritional Information (per 1/4 cup serving):
Calories: 35, Fat: 0g, Carbs: 9g, Protein: 0g

Fruit-Based Treats, Beverages and Herbal Teas for Hydration

Here are the fruit-based treats, beverages and herbal teas with preparation time, cooking time, ingredients, instructions and nutritional information:

Watermelon and Mint Salad

Prep Time: 15 minutes
Cook Time: 0 minutes

Ingredients:
- 4 cups cubed watermelon
- 1/4 cup fresh mint leaves, chopped
- 2 tablespoons lime juice
- 1 tablespoon honey (optional)
- Pinch of salt

Instructions:
1. In a bowl, gently toss together the watermelon, mint, lime juice, honey (if using), and salt.
2. Refrigerate for 30 minutes before serving to allow flavors to blend.

Nutritional Information (per 1 cup serving):
Calories: 46, Fat: 0g, Carbs: 11g, Protein: 1g

Here are 5 fruit-based treatments with preparation time, cooking time, ingredients, cooking instructions, and nutritional values:

Green Smoothie

Prep Time: 5 minutes

Cook Time: None

Ingredients:
- 1 cup unsweetened almond milk
- 1 banana
- 1 cup fresh spinach
- 1/2 cup frozen pineapple chunks
- 1 tbsp chia seeds
- 1 tbsp honey (optional)

Instructions:
1. Add all ingredients to a blender.
2. Blend on high until smooth and creamy.
3. If the smoothie is too thick, add a splash more almond milk to reach desired consistency.
4. Pour into a glass and enjoy immediately.

Nutritional Value (per serving):
Calories: 240, Protein: 5g, Carbs: 47g, Fiber: 9g, Fat: 6g

Baked Apples with Cinnamon and Honey

Prep Time: 10 minutes
Cook Time: 30 minutes

Ingredients:
- 4 apples (e.g., Honeycrisp, Gala, or Fuji)
- 1/4 cup honey
- 1 tsp ground cinnamon
- 1 tbsp butter or coconut oil, melted
- 1/4 cup water or apple juice

Instructions:
1. Preheat oven to 375°F (190°C).
2. Core the apples, leaving the bottom intact to create a cavity.
3. In a small bowl, mix together honey, cinnamon, and melted butter/coconut oil.
4. Stuff the cinnamon-honey mixture into the cavity of each apple.
5. Place the stuffed apples in a baking dish and pour water/apple juice into the bottom.
6. Bake for 25-30 minutes, or until apples are tender when pierced with a fork.
7. Serve warm, drizzled with the liquid from the baking dish.

Nutritional Value (per apple):
Calories: 160, Protein: 1g, Carbs: 38g, Fiber: 4g, Fat: 3g

Lemon and Cucumber Infused Water

Prep Time: 5 minutes
Cook Time: None

Ingredients:
- 1 cucumber, sliced
- 1 lemon, sliced
- 8 cups water
- Ice cubes (optional)

Instructions:
1. In a large pitcher or jar, combine the sliced cucumber and lemon.
2. Pour in the water and gently stir to combine.
3. Refrigerate for at least 2 hours, or up to 24 hours, to allow the flavors to infuse.
4. Serve chilled, with or without ice cubes.

Nutritional Value (per 1 cup serving):
Calories: 5, Protein: 0g, Carbs: 1g, Fiber: 0g, Fat: 0g

Rainbow Fruit Salad

Prep Time: 15 minutes
Cook Time: None

Ingredients:
- 1 cup fresh strawberries, sliced
- 1 cup fresh pineapple chunks
- 1 cup fresh blueberries
- 1 kiwi, peeled and sliced
- 1 orange, peeled and segmented
- 1 tbsp honey (optional)
- 1 tsp lemon or lime juice (optional)

Instructions:
1. In a large bowl, gently combine all the prepared fruits.
2. If desired, drizzle with honey and lemon/lime juice and toss gently to coat.
3. Chill in the refrigerator for at least 30 minutes before serving to allow flavors to blend.

Nutritional Value (per serving):
Calories: 90, Protein: 1g, Carbs: 22g, Fiber: 3g, Fat: 0g

Berry Antioxidant Smoothie

Prep Time: 5 minutes
Cook Time: None

Ingredients:
- 1 cup frozen mixed berries (e.g., strawberries, blueberries, raspberries)
- 1 banana
- 1 cup unsweetened almond milk
- 1 tbsp chia seeds
- 1 tbsp almond butter
- 1 tsp honey (optional)

Instructions:
1. Add all ingredients to a blender.
2. Blend on high until smooth and creamy.
3. If the smoothie is too thick, add a splash more almond milk to reach desired consistency.
4. Pour into a glass and enjoy immediately.

Nutritional Value (per serving):
Calories: 310, Protein: 7g, Carbs: 45g, Fiber: 11g, Fat: 13g

Ginger Lemonade

Prep Time: 10 minutes
Cook Time: 0 minutes

Ingredients:
- 1 cup fresh lemon juice (6-8 lemons)
- 1 cup water
- 2 tablespoons honey or maple syrup
- 2-inch knob of ginger, grated
- Ice cubes

Instructions:
1. In a pitcher, stir together the lemon juice, water, honey/syrup and grated ginger.
2. Add ice cubes and stir well.
3. Optionally, garnish with lemon slices.

Nutritional Information (per 1 cup serving):
Calories: 62, Fat: 0g, Carbs: 16g, Protein: 0g

Green Tea Smoothie

Prep Time: 5 minutes
Cook Time: 0 minutes

Ingredients:
- 1 cup unsweetened green tea, chilled
- 1 banana
- 1 cup fresh spinach
- 1/2 cup frozen mango chunks
- 1 tablespoon almond butter
- 1 tablespoon honey (optional)

Instructions:
1. Add all ingredients to a blender and blend until smooth and creamy.
2. Add more tea or water to reach desired consistency.
3. Sweeten with honey if desired.

Nutritional Information (per serving):
Calories: 265, Fat: 8g, Carbs: 48g, Protein: 6g

Golden Milk Latte

Prep Time: 5 minutes
Cook Time: 5 minutes

Ingredients:
- 2 cups unsweetened almond milk
- 1 teaspoon turmeric powder
- 1/2 teaspoon cinnamon
- 1/4 teaspoon ground ginger
- 1 tablespoon honey or maple syrup
- 1/2 teaspoon vanilla extract

Instructions:
1. In a saucepan, whisk together the milk, turmeric, cinnamon, ginger, honey/syrup and vanilla.
2. Heat over medium, whisking frequently, until steaming hot but not boiling.
3. Remove from heat and use a milk frother to foam the milk if desired.

Nutritional Information (per serving):
Calories: 120, Fat: 3.5g, Carbs: 16g, Protein: 1g

Chamomile Tea

Prep Time: 2 minutes
Cook Time: 5 minutes

Ingredients:
- 1 chamomile tea bag
- 1 cup hot water

Instructions:
1. Bring water to a boil in a kettle or pot.
2. Place tea bag in a mug and pour the hot water over it.
3. Let steep for 5 minutes.
4. Remove tea bag and enjoy!

Nutritional Information (per serving):
Calories: 0, Fat: 0g, Carbs: 0g, Protein: 0g

Peppermint Tea

Prep Time: 2 minutes
Cook Time: 5 minutes

Ingredients:
- 1 peppermint tea bag
- 1 cup hot water

Instructions:
1. Heat water until boiling in a kettle or pot.
2. Place the tea bag in a mug and pour hot water over it.
3. Allow to steep for 5 minutes.
4. Remove tea bag and enjoy!

Nutritional Information (per serving):
Calories: 0, Fat: 0g, Carbs: 0g, Protein: 0g

Hibiscus Tea

Prep Time: 2 minutes
Cook Time: 8 minutes

Ingredients:
- 2 tablespoons dried hibiscus flowers
- 1 cup boiling water
- Honey or agave nectar (optional)

Instructions:
1. Place the dried hibiscus flowers in a teapot or heat-proof pitcher.

2. Pour the boiling water over the flowers.
3. Let steep for 6-8 minutes.
4. Strain the tea into cups.
5. Add honey or agave to sweeten if desired.

Nutritional Information (per 8oz serving, unsweetened):
Calories: 0, Fat: 0g, Carbs: 0g, Protein: 0g

Ginger Turmeric Tea

Prep Time: 5 minutes
Cook Time: 10 minutes

Ingredients:
- 4 cups water
- 1-inch knob fresh ginger, sliced
- 1 teaspoon ground turmeric
- 1 tablespoon honey or maple syrup
- 1 lemon, juiced

Instructions:
1. In a saucepan, combine the water, ginger slices and turmeric.

2. Bring to a boil over high heat, then reduce to a simmer.
3. Simmer for 10 minutes to allow flavors to infuse.
4. Remove from heat and stir in honey/syrup and lemon juice.
5. Strain into mugs and serve hot.

Nutritional Information (per 1 cup serving):
Calories: 32, Fat: 0g, Carbs: 8g, Protein: 0g

28 DAYS MEAL PLAN

FIRST WEEK

Day 1

- Breakfast: Berry and Spinach Breakfast Smoothie
- Lunch: Chickpea Salad
- Dinner: Baked Turmeric Chicken Thighs with Roasted Fingerling Potatoes

Day 2

- Breakfast: Avocado and Smoked Salmon Toast
- Lunch: Lentil Soup
- Dinner: Quinoa Stuffed Bell Peppers

Day 3

- Breakfast: Quinoa Breakfast Bowl
- Lunch: Mediterranean Chicken Skewers with Greek Potato Salad
- Dinner: Sweet Potato and Black Bean Tacos

Day 4

- Breakfast: Buckwheat Pancakes
- Lunch: Veggie and Hummus Wrap
- Dinner: Cauliflower and Chickpea Curry

Day 5

- Breakfast: Veggie & Tofu Scramble
- Lunch: Tofu Stir-Fry
- Dinner: Lemon Herb Chicken with Mashed Cauliflower and Garlic Potatoes

Day 6

- Breakfast: Oatmeal Bowl with Poached Egg Combo

- Lunch: Vegetable and Lentil Shepherd's Pie
- Dinner: Balsamic Glazed Salmon with Roasted Vegetable Buddha Bowl

Day 7

- Breakfast: Smoothie Bowl
- Lunch: Eggplant and Chickpea Curry
- Dinner: Ginger Soy Glazed Pork Chops with Protein-Packed Quinoa Bowl

For Week 2, 3, and 4: Repeat the meal plan from Week 1, adjusting as desired for variety.

INDEX

28 DAYS MEAL PLAN 168
Almond Butter 137
Avocado and Smoked Salmon Toast 58
Avocado Cilantro Lime Sauce 143
Bacon and Cheddar Egg Muffins 46
Baked Apples with Cinnamon and Honey 153
Baked Oatmeal Squares 56
Balsamic Glazed Salmon 124

Balsamic Honey Glaze 147
Balsamic Vinaigrette 138
Beef and Broccoli Stir-Fry 112
Benefits of Adopting an Anti-Inflammatory Diet 13
Berry and Spinach Breakfast Smoothie Packs 60
Berry Antioxidant Smoothie 156
Bircher Muesli 61
Blueberry Almond Overnight Oats 42
Breakfast Burrito 31
Breakfast Burrito Wraps 53
Breakfast Ideas for Meal Preparation 48
Breakfast Muffins 51
Breakfast Muffins Combo 36
Buckwheat Pancakes 27
Cauliflower and Chickpea Curry 99
Chamomile Tea 160
Chickpea Curry 78
Chickpea Salad 80
Chili Lime Shrimp Tacos 135
Chorizo and Egg Breakfast Burrito 68
Coconut Yogurt Parfait 50
Cottage Cheese or Dairy-Free Yogurt Bowl 30
Cucumber Yogurt Sauce 146
Denver Omelet 65

Easy Recipes for Busy Mornings 23
Egg and Veggie Wrap 44
Egg Muffin Cups 48
Eggplant and Chickpea Curry 86
Fluffy Whole Wheat Pancakes 62
Foods and Oils to Avoid 10
Fruit-Based Treats, Beverages and Herbal Teas for Hydration 150
Garlic and Herb Steak 125
Garlic-Herb Yogurt Sauce 144
Ginger Lemonade 157
Ginger Soy Glazed Pork Chops 132
Ginger Turmeric Tea 162
Golden Milk Latte 159
Green Dressing 148
Green Smoothie 152
Green Smoothie with Kale 26
Green Tea Smoothie 158
Greek Potato Salad 131
Guacamole 139
Herb-Roasted Potatoes 122
Herb-Roasted Turkey Breast 118
Hibiscus Tea 162
Honey Mustard Glazed Chicken 119

INTRODUCTION: INFLAMMATION AND ITS IMPACT ON HEALTH 8

Kale and Roasted Vegetable Salad 75

Kitchen Tools and Gadgets for Easy Meal Preparation 15

Lemon and Cucumber Infused Water 154

Lemon Herb Baked Chicken 111

Lemon Tahini Dressing 142

Lemon-Tahini Sauce 146

Lentil and Walnut Meatballs 72

Lentil Soup 83

Mashed Cauliflower and Garlic Potatoes 128

Meal Planning and Preparation 20

Mediterranean Chicken Skewers 121

Mediterranean Quinoa Bowl 74

Mushroom and Spinach Quinoa Pilaf 101

Oatmeal Bowl with Poached Egg 32

Peanut Butter Banana Smoothie Bowl 43

Peppermint Tea 161

Poultry, Meat and Potatoes 110

Protein-Packed Quinoa Bowl 55

Pudding with Berries (Vegan) 96

Quinoa Bowl with Dried Apricots 29

Quinoa Breakfast Bowl 24

Quinoa Stuffed Bell Peppers 88

Rainbow Fruit Salad 155
Roasted Fingerling Potatoes 130
Roasted Red Pepper Pesto 145
Roasted Sweet Potato Wedges 114
Roasted Vegetable Buddha Bowl 82
Sauces, Condiments and Dressings 137
Savory Cheddar Chive Waffles 70
Scrambled Eggs or Tofu with Spinach 23
Shepherd's Pie 115
Smoked Salmon & Cream Cheese 37
Smoothie Packs 49
Spinach and Feta Egg Muffins 45
Spinach and Mushroom Quesadillas 91
Spicy Mango Salsa 149
Steel-Cut Oats with Almond Butter 54
Stuffed Portobello Mushrooms 104
Sweet Potato and Black Bean Hash 127
Sweet Potato and Black Bean Tacos 93
Taco Seasoning 140
The Basics of Anti-Inflammatory Eating 10
The Gut Connection, Inflammatory Responses and Diseases 9
The Role of Diet and Lifestyle 9
Tips for Organizing Your Kitchen Space 18
Tofu Scramble Breakfast Tacos 106

Tofu Scramble Wraps 59
Tofu Stir-Fry 85
Tropical Smoothie Bowl 38
Turmeric Lamb Kabobs 134
Turkey Bacon Avocado Wrap 39
Turkey Meatballs with Zucchini Noodles 116
Tuna Salad Wrap 41
Types of Inflammation 8
Veggie and Hummus Wrap 109
Veggie & Hummus Wrap 28
Veggie & Tofu Scramble 34
Vegetable and Lentil Shepherd's Pie 90
Vegetable Frittata 40
Vegetable Soup 77
Vegetarian and Vegan Options 72
Watermelon and Mint Salad 151
Whole Grain Waffles 33
Zucchini Noodles with Pesto 94

Printed in Poland
by Amazon Fulfillment
Poland Sp. z o.o., Wrocław